M000228892

CENTURY 21
COOK BOOK

DEAR HEALTH-CONSCIOUS FRIEND:

In my forty years practice of pathology, both in the Orient and in the United States, I have seen firsthand the importance of correct diet in the prevention of atherosclerosis. Today, many recognize that the "Western" eating habits of the average person are contributing to this "hardening of the arteries," especially of the heart and brain.

But "Third World" people are also now suffering results from a Western type, rich diet! A study which I conducted on patients treated for "heart attacks" in Bangkok, Thailand, showed an ENORMOUS INCREASE IN CORONARY HEART DISEASE during the past 30 or more years. Whereas in the mid 60's, heart attacks were rare in Thailand (see p. 29), as a result of prosperity which the international influence has brought to this THIRD WORLD CITY, we find three great food factors contributing to the phenomenal increase in heart attack rate:

1. Increased use of red meat and fried foods.
2. Popularization of sweets (e.g. ice cream and pastries).
3. Eating of large, fatty meals late at night (after 7 p.m.).

Research has shown that the atherosclerotic process is reversible.[1,2] It may be retarded by eating a simple diet of natural whole grains, unrefined foods, vegetables, fruits, and by largely eliminating foods of animal origin, high in saturated fats.

In view of these concepts, here are some suggestions:

* Use sparingly fatty foods, especially of animal origin.
* CUT THE PROPORTIONS OF FAT BY HALF, or more, in recipes.
* "SAUTE" by steaming with water, using no oil.
* Use salt sparingly, and eliminate monosodium glutamate.
* Try the "EGGLESS" entree recipes (pp.49-61).
* Use only SKIM milk and cottage cheese.
* Limit desserts to once a week, substituting fruit.
* Seriously consider making breakfast your largest meal.
* Eat simple, light suppers (adults may eliminate entirely).

In the interest of better health and a more productive life, I am sincerely yours,

Ethel R. Nelson, M.D.
Editor

[1,2] Assaad S. Daoud, et al., **Regression of Advanced Atherosclerosis in Swine,** Arch Pathol Lab Med, Vol. 100: 8, July 1976.

Dean Ornish, **Reversibility of Coronary Atherosclerosis,** 61st Scientific Session of the American Heart Assocation, Washington, D.C.

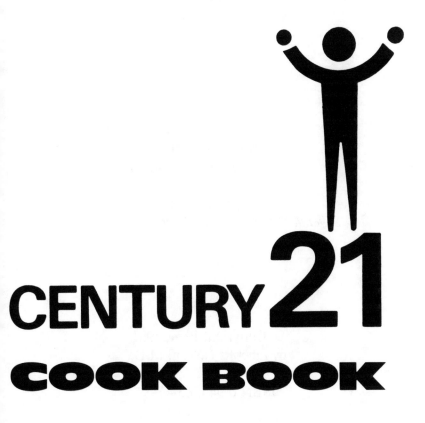

CENTURY 21
COOK BOOK

TEACH Services
Brushton, New York 12916

Revised Edition
(Twenty-fourth Printing)

Approved by the
Seventh-day Adventist Dietetic Association.

ISBN 0-945383-41-X

Published by:

TEACH Services
Route 1, Box 182
Brushton, New York 12916
(518) 358-2125

Table of Contents

CENTURY 21 COOK BOOK

Designed to involve you
in a discovery and
application of advanced
principles of better living.

Foreword

Every now and then a book comes along that is a "must". The **Century 21 Cookbook** is certainly one of them.

Twenty-first century living is here now, whether we want to admit it or not. In fact, changes are occurring so rapidly in all phases of living that it is hard to keep up.

When it comes to the field of medical science and to getting the most out of life physically by having buoyant health and a verve for living we find a brand new emphasis being given to health — namely **PREVENTION.** It is aptly stated by Dr. Ernest L. Wynder, President of the American Health Foundation:

> *"The ultimate answer to the problem of disease is prevention. In simple truth the majority of chronic illnesses and accidents which kill and afflict Americans can be considered preventable. It has become increasingly apparent that treating disease is simply not enough."*

It will be in the field of nutrition that some of our greatest strides in the prevention of disease will yet come. Here preventive medicine reaches its zenith, since food has to do with the very essence of life itself. It is the fuel that maintains, repairs and runs the human machine. It is the source of the material needed to keep the body tissue healthy, vigorous and free of sickness.

Someone has said that the sickness and suffering that everywhere prevail are largely due to popular errors in regard to diet. This is certainly true. We now know that many of the degenerative diseases, such as atherosclerosis (hardening of the arteries), coronary heart disease, high blood pressure, stroke, are due in a large part to our style of living and the kind of food we eat. The very latest information on cancer would indicate that this scourge is definitely influenced by our diet.

We are well aware of the fact that the length of our life span can definitely be influenced by the way we eat, as well as the degree of health that we have while living out our "threescore and ten."

This book will help you learn how to feed your family in such a way that they will enjoy eating the foods that nutritionists tell us are an absolute must if we are going to make it not only through our century but into the twenty-first.

We must increase the fruits, grains and vegetables in the American dietary. There must be a reduction in the amount of highly refined foods such as sugars, cakes, pies, candies, soft drinks and ice cream. There is a definite relationship between a person's personality, if you please, and whether he had a good breakfast or started out with the proverbial cup of coffee and donut.

The very fact that we have so many people who are trying to lose weight is obvious that malnutrition is not limited just to insufficient nourishment. Many times we discover that not only are we overeating, but we are overeating on the wrong foods.

Dr. Ethel Nelson, a physician and homemaker, knows how important the kitchen and food preparation is to the health of the family, the community, and nation.

You will appreciate the discussions before each section of recipes. This information is up to date, concise, and adds greatly to the value of this volume.

Especially helpful are the eggless recipes for those who must control their cholesterol.

Of special interest is the way to prepare vegetable protein foods to take the place of meat. It is now apparent that you can be a well-fed vegetarian, and need not fear short changing your family for lack of a balanced dietary. We congratulate Dr. Nelson and all those who helped compile the **Century 21 Cookbook**. It is practical, easy to read and easy to follow. We feel you will enjoy every page.

J. Wayne McFarland, M.D.
*Co-originator of 5-day
Plan to Stop Smoking.
Fellow of Mayo Clinic
Former teaching faculty and
staff member Dept. of Rehabiliative
Medicine and Dept. of Preventive
Medicine Thomas Jefferson University
School of Medicine,
Philadelphia, Pennsylvania.*

Acknowledgements

Many ladies, and even an occasional man, have had a part in the preparation of this cook book which aims at presenting recipes which are healthful, yet delicious; economical, yet tasty; nutritious, yet meat-free. All the recipes have been tested, not only by those submitting the recipes, but also by many women from several New England communities. The recipes represent the favorites used by a number of homemakers — Louise Anholm, Helen Bond, Frances Crawford, Kathryn Eusey, Jeane Kravig, Ruth Kuester, Rose Lehman, Adele Nelson, Alice Nelson, Frances Read, Joyce Rigsby, Retta Snider, Tanya Stotz, Marvelyn Sturtevant, Donna Toppenberg, Nancy Wall, Cyndee Watts, and Charlene Zeelau.

Miss Donna Morse and Mr. Elvin Kreuger, head dietitians of the New England Memorial Hospital; Mr. Robert Stotz, director of Health Education, New England Memorial Hospital; and Dr. Glenn Toppenberg aided materially in the preparation and compilation of the nutritional capsules found on the divider pages.

Mrs. Florence Silver, who has conducted vegetarian cooking schools for the past fifteen years, besides contributing many of her own recipes, has given invaluable editorial assistance on the book. Calorie calculations were made from "Food Values of Portions Commonly Used," 11th Edition, by Bowes and Church (J. B. Lippincott Co.) and "Nutritive Value of Foods", Home and Garden Bulletin No. 72, U. S. Department of Agriculture. Typing of manuscripts was done by Mrs. Shirley Newmyer and Mrs. Agnes Newton.

— THE EDITOR

high prices and occasional
et shortages at home. But
ain blissfully (perhaps
ly) unaware of privation
e in countries containing
quarter of the population
ld.

rtents for the future say
going to get worse than
now, probably soon and
atastrophically, as Rev.

e time being, the report
he world is going to have
s reliance on North Amer-
supplies. At the same time

ng supplier of feed grains
livestock-grade corn, and
more surprisingly) is the
. 1 exporter of rice

for averting general famine rests
with North America, particularly
the United States.

The United States and Canada
together export something like 90
percent of world soybean exports. It
time in the 1970s could precipitate
famine that would probably wipe
out a sizable share of the 900 million
ultra-poor who live in the world's
40 most "underdeveloped" countries.

Americans, grumbling about 52-
cent bread and $1.49 hamburger, are
aware of high prices and occasional
supermarket shortages at home. But
they remain blissfully (perhaps
dangerously) unaware of privation
and famine

to place its reliance
ican food supplies.

is a leading suppli
including livestock
(perhaps more su
world's No. 1 expor

A single bad
United States and
there is no time t
starvation is to be
crisis is upon us no

More than with
of the world, prin
for averting gen
with North Ame
the United St

What If There Is No Meat?

M. G. HARDINGE, M.D., Dr. P.H., Ph.D.
Former Dean, School of Health
Loma Linda University

LOMA LINDA (EP) — That is a
timely question. However, let us consider
a preliminary one first — What are the
essentials of a good, long-term human
diet?

A diet suitable for the continued
maintenance of health must furnish many
nutrients — maybe 50 or more — in rea-
sonable balance with each other. These

include protein, fat, carbohydrate (starch
and sugar), fiber, minerals, vitamins, together with an adequate intake of water.

No one food provides all of these nutrients, nor is any one foodstuff indis-
pensible. Every country and every pop
ulation group develops its own dietar
pattern based on food availability, cu

Turn to NO MEAT next pag

ispensable ele-
e production of
it is not widely
that modern
— especially ni-
have fuel (pe-
s their raw ma-

ithout fuel as
he propulsion of
chinery large-
iculture simply
carried on with-
ate supplies of
-based fertilizer.
notes that world
hemical fertiliz-

ominously that
rly 1974, there were
signs that many nations —
including some very popu-
lous ones, such as India,
Indonesia, Pakistan and
the Philippines — would
be unable to obtain the
needed amounts of ferti-
lizer regardless of price."

The only way to in-
crease production of
beef — a favorite food in
the more affluent parts of
the world—is to "devise
(A) commercially feasible
means of breeding more
than one calf per cow per
year (and) there does not
appear to be any prospect

ough in
yields acre of soy-
beans" largely because the
soybean "is not very re-
sponsive to nitrogen fertilizer."

Finally, "oceanic fisher-
ies are no longer expand-
ing very rapidly"— in fact
the annual world-wide
catch was down in 1973 by
about 10 percent from the
all-time high of 1970—and
nobody has even a foggy
notion of what kind of
breakthrough will be re-
quired to improve the an-
nual harvest of ocean fish-
es.

Fish is a major article of
many peoples' diet and

Over-p
Sahel be
and def
and other
animals
ground
predicts
ine and r
will be
year is o
ple starv
your hor
— if you
tainment
of thing.

One of
tributors,
R. Brown
of food
only a
will save
throughs

No Meat

Continued from Page 6

tom, preference and prejudice. In western countries where food is abundant, a large proportion of the field crops are fed to animals for conversion to animal products. In countries where food is scarce, the crops are used directly by the people to avoid the great loss incurred in the feeding of great quantities of edible human food to animals for the return of a small amount of meat. Only about 5 per cent of the calories fed to growing beef is returned in the form of meat[1]. The question is how long can we afford to do this? With rapidly decreasing food supplies, it looks as if the meatless diet is the diet of the near future for all nations.

If there is any doubt that a diet without meat can be wholly adequate for human nutrition, we need only look at the population explosion in countries where flesh foods are little used. Take for example a diet that consists largely of rice and dahl (lentils, a legume) as in India; corn, millet, and legumes as in areas of Africa, or bean and corn tortillas as in Latin America[2]. These population groups use little meat, not so much from choice as from necessity. If such dietaries can produce the world's greatest fertility and population growth, there should be no question concerning the adequacy of a western type meatless dietary where the variety of foods to choose from is greater and where milk and eggs are usually available.

That a diet without the use of flesh foods is suitable for human need should really not surprise us since it is well-known that plants are the manufacturers of all primary foods. Only plants have the ability to take materials from the soil and the air and make it into food. No animal organism has this power. Without plant foods, animal life would cease to exist.

Many studies of meatless diets have been reported in recent years with an evaluation of their adequacy in terms of human health. Hardinge and Stare[3] found a close similarity in the food intakes of nonvegetarians and lactoovo vegetarians except for the omission of meat by the latter. Those who used meat had a much higher protein intake, but no benefit was found to acrue from this larger consumption, not even in the growth of the adolescent boys and girls. Nor was there any demonstrable difference between the apparent health of the two groups of pregnant women and their babies.

The longevity and remarkable health of the famous Hunzas is common knowledge. The mainstays of their diets are fruits, nuts, grains, legumes, and vegetables with a little goat milk. Meat, primarily mutton, is eaten only once or twice a year on festive occasions[4]. An examination of 25 old men aged 90 to 110 years by Dr. Paul Dudley White, renowned heart specialist, found them in excellent health. The level of their heart function, blood cholesterol and blood pressures were normal even at that advanced age.

World War II taught us much about the protein values of plant foods. A conclusion drawn from observation of population groups on meatless diets and on the results of experimental studies, led the nutritionists of Harvard University to assure the American people during the war years that the lack of meat need not cause any nutritional deficiency. They said:

". . . as long as this country has access to a plentiful supply of calories and a variety of whole grain cereals and legumes, it is most unlikely that impairment of health from protein deficiency will ever occur"[5].

Then they restated their assurance: "Lumber jacks may demand plenty of red meat to get the timber cut, but the demand rests on habit and not on a nutritional or medical basis."

Dr. Nevin S. Scrimshaw of the Massachusetts Institute of Technology at Cambridge, has recently reviewed the advances in the understanding of protein nutrition[6]. From the results obtained from studies in various countries in the use of mixtures of plant proteins, he concludes that vegetable protein, combined in suitable proportions, have proven as efficient in meeting human needs, even the needs of children, as have animal proteins. He says:

"This knowledge frees us from dependence on the concept of the need for animal protein or amino acids from conventional foods alone." The conventional sources he lists as milk, meat, poultry and eggs. Looking ahead, Dr. Scrimshaw predicts:

"The bulk of present and future needs will be met by conventional plant proteins." These he lists as cereal grains, legumes, (especially soybeans, peanuts, and chick peas), oilseeds and food yeast.

A 1972 report from the Department of Human Nutrition of the Virginia Polytechnic Institute, states that there was no protein deficiency in 7 to 9-year-old girls fed a diet in which cereal grains. and legumes provided nearly all the protein. The diets simulated those of Southern low income families[7].

What, then, if there is no meat? A meatless diet can be wholly adequate for every human need from childhood to extreme old age, and even for the stress of pregnancy and lactation. No longer need anyone fear the day when beef steaks and pork chops will have to give way to the foods of the future — the products of the earth made into tasty dishes with a little milk and probably some eggs.

REFERENCES:

1. Sure, B.: Improving the nutritive value of cereal grains.   J Nutr 50:235, 1953.

2. Jelliffe, D. B.: Child Nutrition in Developing Countries. Public Health Service Publication No. 1822, 1968, pp 17, 28-32.

3. Hardinge, M. G. and Stare, F. J.; Nutritional Studies of Vegetarians. I. Nutritional, physical, and laboratory studies. J Clin Nutr. 2:73, 1954.

4. Toomey, E. G. and White, P. W.: A brief survey of the health of aged Hunzas. Amer Heart J 68:842, 1964.

5. Stare, F. J. and Thorn, G. W.: Some medical aspects of protein foods. Amer J Pub Health 33:1444, 1943.

6. Scrimshaw, N. S.: Nature of protein requirements. J Amer Dietet Assoc 54:94, 1969.

7. Abernathy, R. P., Ritchey, S. J., and Gorman, J. C.: Lack of response to amino acid supplements by preadolescent girls. Amer J Clin Nutr 25: 980. 1972.

PROTEIN PEARLS

What is the daily recommended protein allowance?[1]

- Women   44-48 gms
- Men   52-56 gms
- Children   23-36 gms (increasing requirements with age)

What does protein do in the body?

- Used for building and repairing body tissue
- Utilized for energy only when carbohydrates and fats are not available

What are proteins?

- Proteins are composed of amino acids
- Amino acids that cannot be formed in the bodies of man and animal are called essential amino acids
- Essential amino acids, originally formed by plants, must be present in our daily food
- It is desirable to get protein from a variety of sources

What foods are acceptable sources of protein?

ANIMAL SOURCES
- Meat
- Poultry
- Fish
- Eggs
- Milk
- Cheese

VEGETABLE SOURCES
- Legumes (beans, peas, lentils, garbanzos, soy beans, etc.)
- Nuts (walnuts, pecans, cashews, almonds, etc.)
- Whole grains, especially mixtures, (wheat, rye, oats, corn, rice, barley, millet, etc.)

Do plants provide an adequate protein for the body?

- Plants contain varying amounts of protein
- A mixture of plant foods, eaten in proper amounts, provides an adequate variety of amino acids
- For example: any grain with any legume makes an adequate protein, provided each is in proper amounts

Does a lacto-ovo- vegetarian constantly have to figure out what and how to eat?

- It is not the amino acid content of a single protein source that is important . . .
- But the total supply of amino acids which the whole meal supplies
- IF A DIET HAS ADEQUATE NUTRITIVE CALORIES AND IS COMPOSED LARGELY OF A VARIETY OF UNREFINED FOODS, CHOSEN FROM THE FOUR GENERAL FOOD GROUPS, THE PROTEIN INTAKE IS USUALLY ADEQUATE [2]

ENTREES . . . LEGUMES . . . GRAINS . . . NUTS

What are the advantages of legumes

- High level of protein
- Relatively cheap
- Approximately ten ½ cup servings/pound beans
- Good source of Vitamin B_1
- Good source of iron and phosphorus
- Good source of fiber

Helpful hints on cooking dry beans and peas...[3]

- Soaking beans overnight will shorten the cooking time
- Beans may ferment unless kept cool while soaking
- Cook beans in same water as soaked in
- To soak beans in 1 hour, bring beans to a boil first
- Add salt at END of cooking time as it hardens texture

Varied uses of legumes...

- Soups • Patties • Loaves • Casseroles • Stews • Vegetables • Salads
- Often served with rice or breads — an example of "mix and match" of proteins

What is an example of a concentrated plant protein?

THE SOYBEAN

Why is the soybean unique?

- An acre of land planted in soybeans can produce 10 times as much protein as animals grazing an acre of land [4]
- A pound of beef costs about 4 times as much to produce as a pound of soybean protein
- An excellent source of Thiamine (Vitamin B_1)
- Soybean flour added to wheat bread to the amount of 5% of total flour, makes the protein complete, and also makes the bread more moist and tender
- Soybean flour may be substituted in some entree recipes for the binding qualities of eggs
- Fortified soy "milk" can be safely substituted for cow's milk, especially for infants having a milk allergy

References:
1. Food and Nutrition Board, National Academy of Sciences — National Research Council Recommended Daily Dietary Allowances, Revised 1973
2. Register, U. D., Chairman, Department of Nutrition, Loma Linda University
3. U. S. Dept. of Agriculture Bulletin #326, Pg. 6 & 7
4. The Story Behind Those Meatless "Meats", Popular Science, Oct. 1972

Legumes - Nuts - Grains
(Using Eggs)

PECAN LOAF
213 Cal. per serving

2 Tbsp. margarine — MELT in saucepan.

1 small onion, chopped
1 cup celery, chopped — ADD to margarine and steam for few minutes.

1 tsp. salt
¾ cup milk — ADD and take pan from the heat.

½ cup chopped pecans
1 cup whole wheat bread-
   crumbs
¼ cup chopped parsley
2 eggs, beaten
½ tsp. sage — ADD to other ingredients. Mix well. Bake in oiled pan at 350° for 45 minutes.

SERVES 6

LENTIL AND NUT ROAST
299 Cal. per serving

1 cup lentils, dry — BOIL until done, and liquid is absorbed.

1 egg — BEAT and add to lentils.

½ cup cashews or other nuts — CHOP fine or grind and add to above.

1-13 oz. can evaporated milk
¼ cup salad oil
1½ cup cornflakes
½ tsp. sage
½ tsp. salt — MIX with previous ingredients.
Place in greased baking dish and bake at 350° for 45 minutes.

SERVES 8

GRAPE NUT ROAST
279 Cal. per serving

2 eggs — BEAT eggs.

1 cup Grape Nuts
1½ cups milk
1 tsp. salt
¾ cup chopped nuts
1 Tbsp. chopped onion
1 cup chopped celery
2 Tbsp. margarine — ADD all ingredients to eggs. Let it stand for 20 minutes. Place in greased dish. Bake at 350° for 40 minutes.

SERVES 6

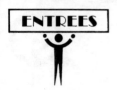

KIDNEY BEAN LOAF

332 Cal. per serving

1 medium onion, chopped fine
2 Tbsp. oil

BROWN onion in oil.

2 cups kidney beans, cooked
1 cup soft bread crumbs
2 eggs, well beaten
2 cups grated cheese
1 Tbsp. tomato catsup

MASH beans and mix ingredients in order. Bake at 350° for 40 minutes.

SERVES 6

PEANUT-BUTTER-CARROT ROAST

310 Cal. per serving

3 cups carrots
1 medium minced onion

PUT through food chopper.

½ cup bread crumbs
2 cups milk
1 cup stewed tomatoes
1 tsp. sage
2 Tbsp. melted butter
1 cup crunchy peanut butter
2 eggs, beaten
1 tsp. salt

MIX remaining ingredients in given order. Pour into baking pan and bake at 350° for one hour. (Smooth peanut butter may be used instead of crunchy, if desired.)

SERVES 8

GARBANZO LOAF

150 Cal. per serving

1 cup cooked garbanzos
1 onion, chopped
¼ cup chopped green
    peppers, or celery or mush-
    rooms (optional)
2 eggs
½ cup tomato soup or milk
1 tsp. Accent
½ tsp. salt

MASH garbanzos and combine all ingredients and bake at 350° for 45 minutes.

SERVES 4

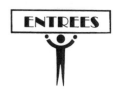

PIMIENTO CHEESE LOAF

288 Cal. per serving

3 pimientos, chopped
½ lb. cream cheese grated
1 egg
2 cups cooked white lima
   beans, mashed
4 Tbsp. onion, chopped
2 Tbsp. parsley, chopped
1 tsp. salt
¾ cup bread crumbs

SERVES 6

MIX and shape into a loaf. Sprinkle with crumbs. Bake in a 325° oven for one hour.

ASPARAGUS LOAF

143 Cal. per serving

½ cup cracker crumbs

ROLL crackers until finely crushed.

2 cups cooked asparagus,
   drained

CUT pieces into 1 inch lengths.

1 cup milk
2 eggs, slightly beaten
2 Tbsp. margarine
1 tsp. salt
1 tsp. grated onion

MIX all ingredients together. Turn into buttered baking dish and bake in moderate oven. Serve with 2 cups of white sauce mixed with ½ cup of chopped parsley.

SERVES 6

SPEEDY OATMEAL HAMBURGERS

115 Cal. per serving

1 cup oatmeal, dry
1 tsp. salt
1 tsp. sage

MIX oats, salt and sage in bowl.

1 medium onion
3 eggs

CHOP onion fine, add to oats. Beat eggs until thick and yellow. Stir oat mixture into eggs quickly and fry in hot oil, just long enough to brown lightly on both sides. Remove at once to warm plate. When all are fried, replace in pan and cover with a tomato-mushroom sauce. Or mix your own by adding a can of mushroom gravy to a can of tomato sauce. Simmer for 20 minutes to ½ hour. Good hot or cold. An alternate sauce, also delicious, is 1 cup of hot water mixed with 1 heaping teaspoon of Vegex. Simmer patties until liquid is mostly absorbed.

SERVES 6

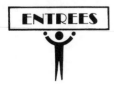

LENTIL PATTIES

96 Cal. per patty

½ lb. dry lentils
1 medium onion, chopped
1 tsp. salt or to taste

COOK together with enough water to cover soaked lentils until lentils are very soft and most of water has been absorbed. (Watch while cooking and add a little more water if lentils get too dry.) Mash lentils, leaving some whole. The electric mixer does this nicely.

4-6 slices day-old bread, cut into ½ inch cubes
1-2 eggs

START with 4 slices of bread and 1 whole unbeaten egg. Stir well into mashed lentils. It should be of a consistency to push from a spoon into pan to form a pattie. More bread may be needed to get right consistency. Flatten with back of spoon. Saute 1 pattie in a mixture of oil and margarine to see if it will stay together. If it breaks apart, add second egg and a little more bread. Saute remaining patties until nicely browned on both sides. Serve with the following sauce:

YIELD: 15 patties

TOMATO SAUCE

7 Cal. per Tbsp.

2½ cups cooked tomatoes
1 Tbsp. sugar
1 tsp. salt

BRING to boil. Thicken as desired with cornstarch paste.

3 Tbsp. cornstarch mixed with
3 Tbsp. water

SERVES 10

OATMEAL-WALNUT PATTIES

209 Cal. per serving

2 eggs
1 cup oatmeal, dry
1 cup ground walnuts (or other kind)
¼ cup evaporated milk
1 medium minced onion
1 tsp. salt
sage if desired
1 Tbsp. soy sauce

BEAT eggs and combine all other ingredients with them. Drop from spoon to form small patties and brown on both sides in hot oil. Cover with gravy, such as cream of mushroom soup thinned with ½ can water, or tomato sauce, or your favorite meatless gravy. Simmer for about ½ hour or bake in oven until hot and bubbly.

SERVES 6

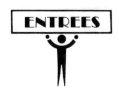

STEAMED PEANUT BUTTER ROAST

263 Cal. per serving

1 cup peanut butter
1 cup flour
1 tsp. salt
1 tsp. sage
1–10 oz. can tomato soup
2 cups water
1 egg
1 small onion, chopped
  (optional)

MIX well. May be made in a blender. Put into greased round tin and steam in a closed kettle over boiling water until set, about 1 hour. Cut in slices. Can be served hot or cold.

SERVES 8

OATMEAL MUSHROOM PATTIES

212 Cal. per serving

1 small potato, grated
2 eggs
1 cup oatmeal, dry

BLEND together, allowing oats to absorb moisture.

1 - 4 oz. can mushrooms
  chopped (save liquid)
1 envelope onion soup mix
2 Tbsp. oil
1 tsp. Accent
½ tsp. sweet basil

DRAIN mushrooms, saving liquid. Mix with oat mixture and shape into patties. Fry in oil until brown. Place in greased casserole.

1 10-oz. can mushroom soup
mushroom liquid, add water
  to ½ cup
1 Tbsp. soy sauce
1 Tbsp. oil

MIX gravy and cover patties in casserole. Bake at 350° for 30 minutes.

SERVES 6

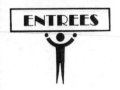

ENTREES

STUFFED PEPPERS

258 Cal. per serving

6 large green stuffing peppers — CUT in half lengthwise and remove all seeds and membranes. Pour boiling water over to cover and let stand for 10 minutes. Remove and drain well.

1 cup rice (do not wash) — TOAST over high heat, stirring constantly until light tan.

2 cups cold water
2 envelopes G. Washington Broth
1/3 cup dehydrated chopped onion
— ADD to rice in pan, bring to boil, cover, turn heat to very low and cook 20-25 minutes.

1 cup ground pecans
1 cup cottage cheese
1 cup Kellogg's Special K
2 eggs
½ cup evaporated milk
2 tsp. chicken style seasoning
¼ cup melted margarine
— MIX well together, and let stand while rice is cooking, then mix with rice mixture.

ARRANGE peppers in 9½" x 13" glass baking dish, stuff with prepared mixture and sprinkle with Italian seasoned bread crumbs.

2-10 oz. cans tomato soup
1 can water
— MIX together or use tomato sauce and pour around peppers. Bake at 350° for 40—50 minutes

SERVES 12

COTTAGE CHEESE PATTIES

217 Cal. per serving

1 cup cottage cheese
1 cup ground cracker crumbs
1 cup chopped walnuts
3 eggs
¼ tsp. sage
¼ tsp. salt
1 finely chopped onion
— MIX all ingredients well. Drop by ice cream scoopfuls or serving spoons on a well greased frying pan. Flatten with spatula and let brown. Turn to brown other side. Place patties in a deep casserole dish.

1-10-oz. can mushroom soup
1 can water
— DILUTE soup with water, or use your favorite gravy. Pour over patties and bake in 350° oven for 20 minutes or until bubbly.

VARIATION: 1 3 oz. pkg. cream cheese may be substituted for cottage cheese to make cream cheese patties.

SERVES 10

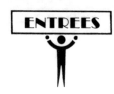

SPINACH COTTAGE CHEESE PATTIES

185 Cal. per serving

1 10 oz. pkg. frozen chopped
  spinach

2 cups cottage cheese
1 cup nuts, chopped
1 small onion, minced
1½ cups herb seasoned
  stuffing, ground
3 eggs

SERVES 10

COOK spinach and drain.

RESERVE ½ cup of crumbs. Combine all remaining ingredients, including the spinach and allow mixture to stand 5 minutes to soften crumbs. Form patties, roll in ground crumbs, and fry until brown on both sides. Serve with brown or mushroom gravy.

MEAT BALLS

135 Cal. per meatball

2 cups cracker crumbs
½ cup nuts
¼ lb. American cheese
1 medium onion

3 eggs, beaten

YIELDS 18 meatballs

GRIND with fine grinder or in blender, or roll with rolling pin.

MIX ground mixture with beaten eggs. Mold into balls. Fry till golden brown (deep fat fryer is best). Simmer meatballs gently for at least an hour in spaghetti sauce of your choice.

COTTAGE CHEESE MEAT BALLS

266 Cal. per serving

1 cup cottage cheese
½ cup wheat germ
½ cup bread crumbs,
  seasoned
1 cup ground pecans
3 eggs
1 large onion, minced

SERVES 6

COMBINE all ingredients. Form into balls. Place in pan. Cover with tomato sauce. Balls will be soft but will set up while baking. Bake one hour at 350°.

HORS D'OEUVRE MEATBALLS

80 Cal. per meatball

1 onion
2 eggs
1 clove garlic

½ cup wheat germ
½ cup bread crumbs
1 tsp. salt
1 Tbsp. parsley
¼ tsp. oregano
½ cup ground pecans

YIELDS: 12 meatballs

BLEND in blender or grate onion and mix with other ingredients.

COMBINE dry ingredients and add the onion egg mixture to it. Add sufficient water to make a stiff mixture. Form into miniature meatballs and brown quickly in hot oil. Remove and drain. Cover with tomato sauce and bake ½ hour at 350°. Serve on toothpicks. May also be made regular size.

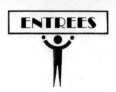

MUSHROOM POTATO POTPIE

327 Cal. per serving

4 cups potatoes, diced
4 carrots, diced
2 stalks celery, diced

BOIL in salted water until nearly done. Reserve water.

2 eggs
2 Tbsp. oil

SCRAMBLE eggs in oil while vegetables are cooking.

1 onion, medium sized
½ cup mushrooms

BREAK up eggs in small bits and add onions and mushrooms.

2 Tbsp. flour
salt to taste
1 Tbsp. chicken style seasoning

ADD flour and seasoning to egg mixture.

3 cups potato water

BLEND in water. Stir smooth. Add more water if necessary to make a medium sauce. Mix vegetables with sauce gently and pour into oiled baking dish. Cover with wheat germ pie crust and bake at 400° till crust is browned.

SERVES 8

WHEAT GERM PIE CRUST

1½ cups sifted flour
2 Tbsp. wheat germ
½ tsp. salt

COMBINE dry ingredients.

½ cup vegetable shortening

CUT shortening into flour until pieces the size of peas.

3 Tbsp. cold water

ADD and mix until dough comes together. Roll on crust.

SPECIAL K ROAST

227 Cal. per serving

1 lb. cottage cheese
2 eggs, beaten
2½ cups Kellogg's Special K
1 onion, chopped
¼ cup chopped pecans
1½ envelope G. Washington Broth
¼ cup melted margarine or oil

MIX all ingredients together and pour into 8 x 8 baking dish. Bake at 325° for 45 minutes covered and 30 minutes uncovered.

SERVES 6

"MEATLESS" MEAT . . .

Canned... Dehydrated... Frozen...

What foods can be used in place of meat?

- Gluten products — made from gluten of flour
- Soybean products
- Nut products

Where did these originate?

- Gluten and soy products have been used in China for many years.
- Textured vegetable protein fiber was developed from a process originating with Boyer, a chemical engineer working for Henry Ford.
- Soybeans are processed to a 90% protein and liquid soy is spun as threads, which give a fibrous texture simulating meat muscle fibers in appearance. By adding different flavors, colors and nutrients, and cutting, cooking and shaping, a final meat-like food is produced. [1]

What are the advantages of commercial vegetable protein foods?

- Low fat, no saturated fat
- No cholesterol
- 40-50% less calories than meat with comparable grams of protein [2] (except fibro-textured proteins which have the same as meat)
- Long Storage life
- Easy to prepare — some may be heated and served as is
- May be used to replace meat in your favorite recipe
- No shrinkage
- Cheaper than meat
- Adds variety to your diet

Available Commercial "Meatless" Meat

	Meat Similarity	Worthington Foods Worthington, OH 43085	La Loma Worthington, OH 43085
CANNED	Steak	Vegesteaks	Swiss steak w/gravy
	Chops	Choplets	Dinner Cuts
	Hamburger	Vegtn. Burger	Vege-burger
	Seasoned		Redi-Burger
	Scallops	Skallops, Veg.	Tender Bits
	Wieners	Vega-links	Linketts
		Super Links	Big Franks
	Sausage	Saucettes	Vegolona
	Chicken	Fri-Chik	Chicken w/gravy
	Turkey	Turkee Slices	
	Nut Roasts	Numete	Nuteena
		Protose	Proteena
	Chili Beans	Chili	
	Sandwich Spread		Sandwich Spread
DRY	Meat Loaf	Granburger	Savory Dinner Loaf
	Meat Patties		Ocean Platter
FROZEN	Chicken	Chik Nuggets	Fried Chicken
		Chicken Slices	
	Beef	Veelets	Savory Meatballs
		Stakelets	Griddle Steaks
	Miscellaneous	Prosage Patties	Corn Dogs
		Fri-Pats	Sizzle Burger

	Meat Similarity	Cedar Lake P.O. Box 8339 Riverside CA 92515
CANNED	Steak	Dinner steaks
	Chops	Chops
	Hamburger	Vegeburger
	Seasoned	Sloppy Joe
	Scallops	Vege-bits
	Wieners	Vegi-Franks
		Tasty-Link
	Sausage	Breakfast Sausage
	Chicken	Chicken Dinner
	Turkey	Terkettes
	Nut Roasts	Nuti-Loaf
	Chili Beans	Chili
	Sandwich Spread	
DRY	Meat Loaf	Burger Granules
	Meat Patties	Beef Patty Mix
		Chicken Patty Mix

Something Better Products

Imt. Cheese Sauce
Imt. Cheese Spread
Imt. Pimento Cheese
3 Grain Pecan
7 Grain Burger

Commercial Meat Alternates

MOCK MEAT LOAF (Eggless)
329 Cal. per serving

1-20 oz. can meatless burger*
1 cup oatmeal, dry
1 cup dry bread crumbs
1 cup ground nuts
1 ground onion
1-10 oz. can mushroom soup
garlic and salt to taste

MIX all together and mold into a loaf, placing it in a well greased pan.

2 Tbsp. water
2 Tbsp. oil

MIX and baste loaf. Bake until brown and firm at 350°.

SERVES 8

HOLIDAY LOAF
308 Cal. per serving

1/4 cup margarine (1/2 stick)
1 medium chopped onion

SAUTE the onion in margarine.

1 pkg. G. Washington Broth
1 tsp. chicken style seasoning

ADD seasonings and broth.

1/2 cup chopped nuts
3 eggs
1/4 cup milk
1 pint cottage cheese
2 1/2 cups Kellogg's Special K
1-13 oz. can Soyameat chicken style, diced

COMBINE with other ingredients. Bake in greased loaf pan, 1 - 1 1/2 hours at 350°.

SERVES 8

BURGER ROAST (Eggless)
270 Cal. per serving

1-20 oz. can meatless burger*
1 cup walnuts, chopped
1 cup onion, ground
1/4 cup oil
1/4 cup oatmeal, dry

MIX all ingredients together. Place in oiled baking dish.

3 bay leaves

2 cups boiling water
1/2 tsp. Savorex

SCATTER bay leaves over the top.

COVER roast with boiling water in which the Savorex has been dissolved. Bake covered at 425° for 30 minutes and 325° for one hour. Open to brown a few minutes.

*See pg. 61

SERVES 8

— 21 —

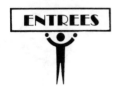

ENTREES

QUICK BURGER LOAF (Eggless)   165 Cal. per serving

2 cups meatless burger*
2 Tbsp. flour, soy or wheat
½ pkg. onion soup mix

MIX together thoroughly. Be sure to mix the onion soup before taking out half of it.

½ cup evaporated milk

ADD and mix well. Place in well greased loaf pan, and bake at 350° for 45 minutes.

SERVES 6

VITA-BURGER LOAF *(pictured on cover)*   186 Cal. per serving

1 cup Vita-Burger
1 cup hot water

COMBINE and let stand 10 minutes.

1 medium potato

PEEL and grate into Vita-Burger.

1 medium diced onion
2 Tbsp. oil

SAUTE onion in oil and add to other ingredients.

3 eggs
½ cup ground pecans
¼ cup wheat germ

ADD and mix thoroughly. Place in well greased loaf pan and bake at 350° about 40 minutes. Unmold and serve with tomato sauce.

SERVES 8

PECAN BURGER LOAF (Eggless)   240 Cal. per serving

2 Tbsp. oil
1 small minced onion

SAUTE the onion in oil.

¼ cup chopped parsley
1 cup chopped celery
½ cup meatless burger*

ADD to onions and stir well.

1 envelope G. Washington
   Broth
½ tsp. salt
1¼ cups milk

ADD and mix well.

½ cup chopped pecans
1 cup whole wheat bread
   crumbs
2 Tbsp. soy flour

COMBINE and add to other ingredients. Mix well. Pour into a well greased baking pan. Bake at 375° for 25 min. Remove from oven. Stir loaf well and return to oven for 20 min. longer until nicely browned on top.

*See pg. 61

SERVES 6

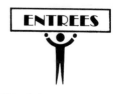

CHOPLET WALNUT ROAST

337 Cal. per serving

1 cup walnuts 1-20 oz. can Choplets (see pg. 61) 1 onion 1½ cups bread crumbs	GRIND all together.
¼ cup oil 3 eggs	Add to above mixture. Mix well. Bake 450° for 45 minutes.

SERVES 8

MOCK TUNA (Eggless)

1-13 oz. can Soyameat, fried chicken style	DRAIN and grate coarsely.
1 small can Tartex 1 small onion, diced ½ cup diced celery ½ cup mayonnaise	ADD to soyameat and mix thoroughly. If desired, additional salt may be added.

MOCK SALMON LOAF (Eggless)

Use above recipe but add 1 cup bread crumbs, and 1 tsp. paprika. Pack into well greased pan or mold, and bake at 350° for 45 minutes.

CASHEW BURGER CASSEROLE (Eggless)

348 Cal. per serving

1-20 oz. can meatless burger* 1 cup diced celery 1 cup chopped cashews ½ cup cooked brown rice 2-10 oz. cans mushroom soup ½ cup water ¼ cup oil	COMBINE all ingredients and mix well. Pour into greased casserole and bake one hour at 350°.

SERVES 8

*See pg. 61

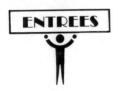

ZUCCHINI CASSEROLE (Eggless)

289 Cal. per serving

1½ lb. zucchini squash (about 6 cups)	SLICE. Cook 2-3 minutes. Drain well. Place half in the bottom of a greased baking dish.
1-20 oz. can meatless burger* 1 medium onion, chopped ¼ cup oil	SAUTE burger and onion in oil until browned. Pour over squash in dish.
1 cup instant rice 1 tsp. garlic salt 1 tsp. oregano	SPRINKLE uncooked rice and seasonings over the burger.
2 cups cottage cheese	SPOON over the rice, and cover with remaining squash.
1-10 oz. can mushroom soup	SPREAD over top.
1 cup grated mild cheese	SPRINKLE on top. Bake at 300° for 35-40 minutes.

SERVES 10

CREAMED CHIPPED BEEF (Eggless)

186 Cal. per serving

4 oz. Soyameat, beef style	CUT or tear into small pieces.
4 Tbsp. oil	SAUTE in oil until lightly browned.
3 Tbsp. flour	ADD flour and mix well.
2 cups milk	ADD milk gradually, stirring constantly. Cook and stir over medium heat until thickened. May be served over toast cups, toast slices, pancakes, waffles or biscuits for breakfast. For lunches
SERVES 6	or suppers, serve on baked potatoes.

QUICKIE MACARONI CASSEROLE (Eggless)

230 Cal. per serving

3½ to 4 cups cooked macaroni 2 cups cottage cheese 2 cups Italian tomato sauce, see page 32 ½ cup chopped olives or 1 4 oz. can 1 cup meatless burger* (optional)	COMBINE in casserole. Soy omelette (pg. 115) can be substituted for the cottage cheese. May be stored in refrigerator and baked the next day at 350° for one hour or bake at 350° for 45 minutes.

SERVES 6

*See pg. 61

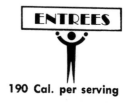

GOURMET CASSEROLE (Eggless)

190 Cal. per serving

2 cups cooked rice
2 cups diced chicken style
  Soyameat
1 10 oz. can mushroom soup
½ cup milk
½ cup soy "mayonnaise"
½ tsp. salt

MIX well first six ingredients.

1 cup celery, chopped
½ cup onion, chopped
1 4 oz. can mushrooms

SAUTE celery, onions and mushrooms and add to rice mixture. Place in greased 2 quart casserole.

¼ cup slivered almonds
paprika

SPRINKLE the top with almonds and paprika. Bake at 350° for 40 minutes.

SERVES 10

MILLET OR RICE MUSHROOM CASSEROLE (Eggless) 288 Cal. per serving

1 cup raw millet or rice

TOAST in dry frying pan until lightly browned.

1 onion, chopped
1 - 4 oz. can mushrooms,
  chopped
1 20 oz. can meatless burger*
4 Tbsp. oil

SAUTE in oil.

1 10 oz. can mushroom soup
4 cups water
½ cup sunflower seed
  (optional)
½ tsp. garlic salt
½ tsp. seasoned salt

ADD remaining ingredients, mixing well. Pour into greased casserole dish and bake at 350° for one hour.

SERVES 8

ALMOND BAKE SOYAMEAT (Eggless)

360 Cal. per serving

1 13 oz. can Soyameat,
  chicken style, chopped
2 cups thinly diced celery
½ cup slivered almonds
½ tsp. salt
2 Tbsp. grated onion
1 cup soy "mayonnaise"
2 Tbsp. lemon juice
1 5½ oz. can Chinese noodles

COMBINE all ingredients and put into casserole dish.

1 cup grated mild cheese

TOP with grated cheese. Bake at 450° 10-15 minutes. This is good and quick.

SERVES 8

*See pg. 61

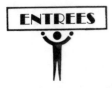

ONE DISH MEAL (Soyameat and Rice) (Eggless)   302 Cal. per serving

1 medium onion, diced
1 cup diced celery
1 cup rice, uncooked
1 cup Soyameat, chicken
   style (diced)
1 cup carrots, diced

MIX onion, celery, rice, carrots and Soyameat together and put into casserole.

1/3 cup oil
1 tsp. Vegex
2 cups water
3 pkgs. G. Washington Broth
1 can mushroom soup

PUT oil, Vegex, water, broth and soup into saucepan and cook for 3 minutes. Pour sauce over casserole and mix gently. Bake 350° for one hour.

SERVES 6

CABBAGE ROLLS (Eggless)   331 Cal. per serving

1 cup rice
1½ cups water
1 tsp. salt

COOK rice in water with salt added.

¾ cup bread crumbs
½ cup brewer's yeast
2 Tbsp. soy sauce
½ cup oatmeal, dry
1-20 oz. can meatless burger*
1 clove garlic, chopped
¼ cup oil

MIX with rice in bowl until well blended.

Grated cheese, chopped hard boiled eggs or chopped nuts can be substituted for the burger.

1 head cabbage

WILT cabbage until leaves can be easily removed, by cutting out core and steaming in small amount of water. Separate leaves. Put 2-3 Tbsp. of mix in each cabbage leaf. Fold ends of leaves to middle, then roll up and secure with toothpicks.

1 pkg. onion soup mix
5 cups hot water

MIX to make a broth. Pour over cabbage rolls placed in electric fry pan or in pan in oven at 350°. When most of moisture is absorbed, after about 30 minutes, add tomato or mushroom sauce and continue cooking another 10 minutes.

SERVES 8

MOCK CHICKEN STEW (Eggless)   206 Cal. per serving

2 carrots cut to bite size
½ onion, chopped
½ cup cashews
5 slices of Soyameat chicken
   style, torn to bite size
chicken style seasoning to
   taste

COMBINE in kettle. Cover with water and cook slowly one hour. Just before serving thicken broth with cornstarch.

SERVES 4

*See pg. 61

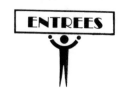

POTPIE (Eggless)

226 Cal. per serving

1 potato, cubed
2 carrots, sliced
1 stalk celery, diced
¼ cup diced onion
¼ cup lima beans
1 tsp. salt

COOK vegetables until almost tender in ¼ cup water.

1 13 oz. can chicken style
Soyameat (diced)
1 10 oz. can mushroom soup

ADD soyameat (including liquid) and mushroom soup. Pour into 9x9 baking dish.

½ recipe pie crust

TOP with pie crust. Bake at 425° for 30 minutes.

SERVES 8

Small amounts of other vegetables may be added if desired.

STUFFED TOMATOES (Eggless)

202 Cal. per serving

8 medium sized tomatoes

SCOOP out tomato pulp, and drain shells. Chop pulp.

½ cup meatless burger*
1½ cups cooked brown rice
1 small chopped onion
½ tsp. salt
1 Tbsp. olive oil

MIX with tomato pulp. Fill tomato shells. Bake at 350° for 30 minutes.

VARIATION: Use this to stuff peppers or onions, using 1 cup of tomato sauce for tomato pulp.

SERVES 4

WALNUT CROQUETTES (Eggless)

185 Cal. per serving

1 small onion, chopped
½ cup celery, chopped
1 - 4 oz. can mushrooms,
chopped
1 cup gluten bits* chopped

SAUTE onion, celery, mushrooms and Vegebits in small amount of oil.

1 cup walnuts, chopped
2 cups rice, cooked
½ cup herb-seasoned stuffing
½ 10 oz. can mushroom soup
3 Tbsp. flour
1 tsp. soy sauce

COMBINE all ingredients and shape into croquettes. Roll in cracker crumbs, rolled corn flakes or additional finely ground stuffing. Place on greased sheet and bake at 350° for 20-30 minutes. Serve with gravy of choice.

SERVES 10

*See pg. 61

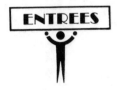

MOCK CHICKEN CROQUETTES

255 Cal. per serving

1 pound chicken style Soyameat 4 hard cooked eggs	GRIND coarsely.
1 cup water ½ cup Cream of Wheat, dry	BOIL water and stir cereal into it. Cook until very thick. It should make ¾ cup. Add to soyameat.
2 Tbsp. margarine 1 tsp. onion powder 3 Tbsp. evaporated milk ⅛ tsp. salt 2 tsp. chicken style seasoning	ADD and mix all ingredients well. Shape into croquettes. Bread and brown in a little oil.

SERVES 8

OATBURGERS (Eggless)

174 Cal. per serving

1-20 oz. can meatless burger* 2 cups oatmeal, dry 1 minced onion 1-10 oz. can mushroom soup 1 tsp. Italian seasoning	MIX all together and form into patties. Place on oiled cookie sheet and bake at 350° until brown. Turn once to brown the other side. Serve with tomato sauce or your favorite gravy.

SERVES 8

CASHEW NUT PATTIES

247 Cal. per serving

2 eggs 1 medium onion 1 Tbsp. soy sauce 1 Tbsp. oil ½ cup milk 1½ cups cashews 1 clove garlic 1 tsp. paprika	WHIZ in blender until smooth.
½ tsp. celery salt 1 tsp. salt 1 tsp. poultry seasoning ¾ cup meatless burger* 1 cup oatmeal, dry	COMBINE and let stand a few minutes. Fry as patties and put in a large 9x13 baking dish. Put a dash of soy sauce on each patty and cover with 1 to 1½ cups water. Cover and bake at 400° for 30 minutes. Add favorite gravy and serve. May be made ahead of time and after baking store in refrigerator or freezer. Then, before serving, add gravy and bake covered until heated through.

SERVES 8

*See pg. 61

Fascinating Foreign Facts

The incidence of coronary heart disease is strikingly
less or absent among...

- Thais (Thailand) who eat rice, fish, vegetables with little red meat or dairy products [1]
- Italians who use unsaturated olive oil in preparation of food
- Japanese (in Japan) with 13% fat content of diet have an average serum cholesterol of 120 mg/dl
  - Hawaiian Japanese with 32% fat in diet have 4 times as many coronaries and average cholesterol of 183

CONTRAST

  - U. S. Japanese eating a 45% fat diet with 10 times more coronaries, have average cholesterol of 213 [2]
- Korean Buddhist monks and nuns living on rice, soybeans, vegetables and fruit

Sample World cross-section of Vegetarians... [3]

North China peasants eat adequately a millet-corn-soy-bean mixture

Otomi Indians of Central Mexico eating tortillas, beans, peppers and local foods have no obesity or high blood pressure

Japanese Buddhist monks enjoy good health eating rice, barley, soy products, vegetables and rapeseed oil

Northern Indian tribes eating grains, legumes, vegetables, fruit and milk have superior health & physique

Yemenite Jews eating predominantly vegetarian diet have significantly lower cholesterol blood levels than other Israelis

Lacto-vegetarian Belgian monks have significantly lower blood cholesterol than omnivorous Benedictine monks whose diet is similar to the average American man

Longevity especially reported among...

Okinawans eating non-flesh native diet

Hunzas (Kashmir) eating a predominantly vegetarian-fruit-grain diet [4]

Vilcabambans (Ecuador) living on a low-calorie vegetarian diet [5]

Seventh-day Adventists in California survey

Fat Facts . . .

> "Coronary Heart Disease has reached enormous proportions, striking more and more at younger subjects. It will result in coming years in the greatest epidemic mankind has faced unless we are able to reverse the trend by concentrated research into its cause and prevention."—Executive Board, World Health Organization, 1969

What causes coronary heart disease (CHD)?

- Fatty materials (mostly cholesterol) accumulate in the walls of the coronary arteries, blocking the heart's blood supply

What are the greatest risk factors in CHD?

- Habitual diet high in saturated (solid) fats
- High blood lipids (cholesterol and triglycerides)
- Family history of CHD in early life (prior to age 50)
- High blood pressure
- Cigarette Smoking
- Obesity
- Diabetes mellitus
- Sedentary living

Will modifying the diet prevent CHD?

- Change from a high to a low cholesterol diet has resulted in decrease in size of fatty deposits in arteries of experimental animals

What practical improvement in diet can be made?

LIMIT: Meat, especially organ meats (e.g. liver), whole milk, cheese from whole milk or cream, solid shortening, butter, egg yolks (single highest source of cholesterol), excessive sweets (sucrose raises triglyceride level)

USE: Grains, nuts, legumes, vegetables and fruit (low fat, no saturated fat, no cholesterol) [6] (See pg. 48 also)

What age groups should alter the diet?

- A life-long diet producing a lowered serum cholesterol level will retard development of CHD. Such a diet is recommended for entire populations, including children and adolescents [7]

References:
1. Stitnimankarn, T. et. al, Autopsy Findings in the Aged Population of Thailand, Arch Path 88: August 1969
2. Fat of the Land, Time, Vol. 77, Jan 13, 1961, pg. 48-52
3. Hardinge, M. G. and Crooks, H., Non-Flesh Dietaries, J. Am. Diet. Assoc. 43; Dec. 1963
4. Leaf, A., Every Day is a Gift When you are Over 100. Nat'l Geographic 154:93-119, 1973
5. Davies, D., A Shangri-la in Ecuador, New Scientist 57: 236-237, 1973
6. Report of Inter-Society Commission for Heart Disease Resources, 1972
7. Atherosclerosis, Medical World News, April 17, 1970

Foreign

SOYACHIK TETRAZZINI

298 Cal. per serving

4-oz. thin spaghetti

BREAK spaghetti in 2 inch pieces and cook until tender, drain.

1 cup diced Soyameat
    chicken style
1-10 oz. can mushroom soup
½ cup milk
¼ cup pimento, chopped
¼ cup green pepper, minced
1 small onion, minced
1 cup shredded mild cheese

COMBINE spaghetti with remaining ingredients, reserving half of the cheese to sprinkle on top of mixture. Place in a 1½ quart oiled casserole. Bake at 400° for 30 minutes.

SERVES 4

BAKED BEANS ALLA ROMANA (Eggless)

230 Cal. per serving

2 1 lb. cans cannellini beans
1 medium onion, thinly sliced
1 clove crushed garlic
2 Tbsp. minced parsley
¼ tsp. dried basil
1 cup tomato sauce
¼ cup chopped ripe olives
2 Tbsp. olive oil

COMBINE all ingredients in a covered casserole and bake at 325° for 1 hour. Sprinkle with grated cheese if desired and bake uncovered until cheese browns.

VARIATION: Try this with chick peas.

SERVES 6

SOY CHICKEN CACCIATORE (Eggless)

172 Cal. per serving

2 medium onions, chopped
1 green pepper, chopped
olive oil to cover bottom of pan

COOK in oil until soft.

1 pint tomato sauce
1 tsp. garlic powder
1 tsp. oregano
¼ tsp. thyme, optional

ADD and simmer covered about 15 minutes.

1-13 oz. can Soyameat, fried
    chicken style

BREAK with a fork into bite sized pieces, and add to sauce. Simmer another 15 min. Serve over hot rice or spaghetti.

SERVES 6

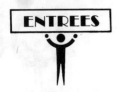

ITALIAN TOMATO SAUCE

147 Cal. per cup

2 Tbsp. olive oil
1 or 2 cloves minced garlic

SAUTE garlic in oil.

1 quart tomatoes

STRAIN or puree in blender and add to oil.

1-6-oz. can tomato paste
1 bay leaf
2 tsp. salt
½ tsp. oregano
½ tsp. basil
1 tsp. sugar (optional)

ADD to sauce and simmer until thick.

VARIATION: Sliced onions may be sauteed with the garlic.

SPANISH TOMATO SAUCE

Use above recipe, adding 1 cup chopped onions and ½ cup diced green pepper. For a Mexican flavor, add 1 tsp. cumin to the sauce.

EGGPLANT PARMIGIANA (Eggless)

335 Cal. per serving

1 medium eggplant
oil

PEEL eggplant, if desired. Slice crosswise in ¼ inch slices. Brush lightly with oil.

seasoned dry bread crumbs

DIP each slice in bread crumbs or breading mixture. Bake on oiled cookie sheet in 400° oven, turning once when brown. Delicious when eaten as is.

Italian tomato sauce
½ pound mozzarella cheese

POUR some tomato sauce to cover the bottom of baking dish. Alternate layers of baked eggplant, tomato sauce and mozzarella cheese. Bake at 350° about ½ hour.

SERVES 6

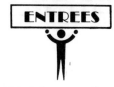

LASAGNA

434 Cal. per serving

1 lb. lasagna noodles

COOK noodles as directed on package with 1 tbsp. salt and 1 tbsp. oil added to the water.

1 lb. ricotta cheese
1 egg, optional

COMBINE the cheese with the egg and mix well.

1 lb. shredded mozzarella cheese
1 quart Italian tomato sauce

ASSEMBLE lasagna by alternating layers as follows: cover bottom of pan with tomato sauce, then noodles, ½ of ricotta cheese mixture, ¼ of mozzarella, additional sauce. Repeat with noodles and cheeses, ending with a layer of noodles on top. Sprinkle the remaining mozzarella and sauce on top. Bake at 350° about 30 minutes.

SERVES 10

VARIATION: Meatless burger may be sauteed in oil and used in between the layers.

SPINACH LASAGNA

402 Cal. per serving

10-oz. pkg. frozen chopped spinach

COOK according to directions and drain.

1 lb. lasagna noodles

COOK according to directions on package. Drain and rinse with cold water.

1 medium onion, chopped
½ green pepper, chopped
3 Tbsp. oil

SAUTE onion and pepper in oil for 5 minutes.

2 - 1 lb. cans of tomatoes
6-oz. can tomato paste
1 Tbsp. oregano flakes
1 bay leaf
½ tsp. salt
¼ cup fresh parsley, chopped

ADD tomato paste and tomatoes to onions. Break up larger tomato pieces. Add seasonings and simmer 30 minutes.

1 lb. cottage cheese
8 oz. mozzarella cheese, cubed
½ cup Parmesan cheese
1 egg

ADD cheeses and egg to chopped spinach and mix well. Cover bottom of 9x13 inch baking dish with one third of tomato sauce. Cover with 1/3 the noodle strips, half the spinach mixture and half of mozzarella. Spread one third more of tomato sauce and repeat layer as before. Top with noodles and remaining tomato sauce. Sprinkle with Parmesan cheese. Bake at 350° 40 minutes.

SERVES 10

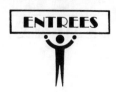

ENTREES

LUIGI'S PIZZA (Eggless)

227 Cal. per slice

1 pkg. yeast 1-2/3 cups warm water	SPRINKLE yeast over water to dissolve.
2 cups whole wheat flour 2 cups unbleached white flour 1½ tsp. salt 1 Tbsp. oil, optional	ADD and turn out on board with additional flour as needed to knead. Roll out to fit a large, greased pan. Let rise while preparing the sauce.
1 large can plum tomatoes	STRAIN; spread out over pizza dough.
1 Tbsp. olive oil ½ tsp. oregano ¼ tsp. garlic salt	SPRINKLE over top. Bake at 350° for 15 minutes. Remove from oven.
8 oz. mozzarella cheese mushrooms, peppers, onions 12 slices	SHRED and put on top of half baked pizza. At this time you could also add sauted mushrooms, peppers or onions to taste. Bake 15-20 minutes longer.

QUICKIE COTTAGE CHEESE PIZZA (Eggless)

114 Cal. per slice

6 slices whole wheat bread 1½ cups Italian tomato sauce	SPREAD on cookie sheet. Spread tomato sauce over each slice.
mushrooms, olives, onions, etc.	MAY be spread over tomato sauce.
1 - 4 oz. can chopped olives	SPREAD evenly over topping.
1 pint cottage cheese	SPREAD generously over olives. Bake at 350° for 20-30 minutes until cottage cheese begins to melt.

PASTA VERDE (Eggless)

351 Cal. per serving

8 oz. spaghetti or linquine or noodles	COOK in boiling water.
2/3 cup boiling water 1 - 3 oz. pkg. cream cheese	MIX together.
2 Tbsp. sweet basil 4 Tbsp. chopped parsley 1 clove minced garlic ⅛ cup olive oil salt to taste	ADD and mix well. When noodles are tender, toss with the sauce, heap on a platter and surround with vegetarian meatballs. (See pg. 17)

SERVES 4

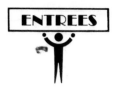

CORN MEAL TORTILLAS

84 Cal. per tortilla

½ cup yellow cornmeal
½ cup cold water

MIX together.

1 cup boiling water
1 tsp. salt

STIR cornmeal mixture into salted boiling water. Keep stirring over the heat until thick. Remove from heat and put in a bowl.

¼ cup oil

ADD and mix thoroughly.

1 cup whole wheat flour
1 cup unbleached white flour

STIR in gradually to make a soft dough. Use additional flour to knead. Knead till smooth. Divide into 18 equal portions. Roll each into a ball. Flatten, and roll out thin on a floured board. Bake on a hot ungreased skillet until lightly browned on both sides.

YIELD: 18 tortillas

WHEAT TORTILLAS

103 Cal. per tortilla

3 cups whole wheat flour
1 tsp. salt

STIR flour before measuring and combine with salt.

1/3 cup oil
1 cup water

BEAT with a fork and add to flour, stirring to moisten evenly. Divide into 18 portions. Roll or pat into thin circles about 5 inches in diameter. Bake on a hot ungreased skillet or grill till lightly browned on both sides.

YIELD: 18 tortillas

ENCHILADAS (Eggless)

243 Cal. per Enchilada

18 tortillas

MAKE as above or use the packaged variety. The above are soft enough to roll. If packaged kind is stiff, dip in hot tomato sauce before rolling.

1 large onion, chopped
3 cups meatless burger*
½ cup oil
1 - 2 cloves minced garlic
½ cup chopped olives, optional

SAUTE all until brown, about 10 minutes. Place about 2 Tbsp. of filling on each tortilla and roll up.

1 quart Spanish tomato sauce

USE your favorite sauce or see page 32.
Cover bottom of baking dish with sauce. Place rolled tortillas seam side down in tomato sauce. Cover with more sauce.

1 medium onion, chopped
1 cup grated mild cheese

SPRINKLE on top of tortillas. Bake at 350° about 30 minutes.

18 Enchiladas

*See pg. 61

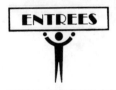

ENTREES

BEAN TORTILLAS

163 Cal. per tortilla

1 cup dry pinto beans

SOAK overnight and then cook in same water, until tender. Drain.

1-10 oz. can tomato soup
1 tsp. onion salt

ADD to beans and heat through.

12 tortillas
salad greens
onions
chopped parsley

FOLD tortillas in half. Fill partially with bean mixture. Add shredded greens and chopped onions. Good also with chopped fresh tomatoes and shredded cheese.

12 tortillas

SPANISH BROWN RICE

361 Cal. per serving

¼ cup olive oil
1 medium onion, chopped
1 small diced green pepper
1 clove minced garlic

SAUTE in a heavy pan for just a few minutes. They should not brown.

1 cup canned tomatoes or
sauce
1 Tbsp. salt
2 cups brown rice, raw
4 cups water

BOIL rapidly for 5 minutes then turn heat down to simmer about 45 minutes. Turn the heat off, and let stand about 10 minutes to absorb all the liquid.

2 pimentos
½ cup olives

SLICE olives and pimentos and decorate top of rice.

SERVES 6

SPANISH LENTILS

272 Cal. per serving

3 cups cooked lentils
2 cups stewed tomatoes
3 Tbsp. oil
1 onion, chopped
1 green pepper, chopped
1 tsp. soy flour
1 tsp. salt
3 Tbsp. food yeast
1 tsp. oregano
1 tsp. ground celery seeds

COMBINE all ingredients and cook until thoroughly heated. Delicious served plain or over rice.

SERVES 6

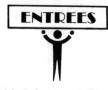

TAMALE PIE

219 Cal. per serving

1 cup milk **1 tsp. salt**	HEAT just up to boiling.
¾ cup corn chips	COMBINE with hot milk and stir until smooth.
12 ripe olives, sliced **1 egg, slightly beaten** **1½ cups corn niblets**	ADD and mix thoroughly.
1 chopped onion **½ cup chopped green pepper** **2 Tbsp. oil**	SAUTE onion and pepper in oil.
2 cups stewed tomatoes **pinch of garlic salt**	ADD to onions and peppers and bring to a boil. Combine with corn mixture and pour into a casserole. Bake at 350° for 30 minutes.

SERVES 6

MEXICAN CHILI

258 Cal. per serving

1 cup dried kidney or pinto beans	SOAK beans overnight; cook until tender.
¼ cup oil **½ clove garlic, finely chopped** **¾ cup onions, finely chopped** **½ cup green pepper, finely ground** **½ cup celery, finely chopped**	BROWN garlic, onions, pepper, celery in hot fat in skillet, or also can be simmered in water, without any oil.
20 oz. can meatless burger*	ADD meatless burger and fry till slightly brown.
½ tsp. paprika **1 tsp. cumin (optional)** **1½ tsp. salt** **2½ cups canned tomatoes** **#2 can**	ADD seasonings, tomatoes and cooked beans, including liquid. Simmer.

SERVES 8

*See pg. 61

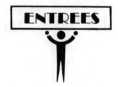

ENTREES

GREEK STUFFING

334 Cal. per serving

1 large onion, chopped
¼ cup oil

SAUTE onion in oil.

1 cup raisins, seedless
1 cup or less walnuts, chopped
   or roasted chestnuts or
   pine nuts

ADD raisins, walnuts and other nuts if available. Set aside, covered to soften raisins.

¾ cup rice, uncooked
1-20 oz. can meatless burger*

COOK rice, add rice and burger. Serve with cranberry jell or sauce. Bake 350° for 20-30 minutes.

SERVES 8

DIETER'S QUICHE LORRAINE

195 Cal. per serving

LOW CALORIE PIE CRUST

(75 Cal. per serving)

½ cup flour
⅛ tsp. salt
1 Tbsp. oil
4 Tbsp. cold water

MIX all together in order given. Knead until pastry forms a ball. Chill well in refrigerator before rolling out on a lightly floured board. Place in a 9 inch pie pan. Prick the bottom in several places with a fork and quick brown in a 425° oven about 10 minutes.

FILLING

1 Tbsp. bacon flavored soy bits
½ cup chopped Swiss or
   mild cheese

SPRINKLE on the bottom of the pie crust.

3 eggs

BEAT on high speed in blender until frothy.

1 cup skim milk
½ cup low fat cottage cheese

ADD to blender and whiz until smooth.

2 Tbsp. dried parsley
2 Tbsp. dried onion flakes

STIR in. Pour mixture into the pie crust.

1 Tbsp. bacon flavored soy
   bits

SPRINKLE on top. Bake at 325° for 45 minutes.

SERVES 6

Less than 200 calories per serving.

*See pg. 61

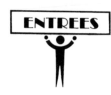

SYRIAN BREAD SANDWICH (Eggless)   Filling: 166 Cal. per serving

**1 - 1 lb. can garbanzos
   (mashed with fork)**
¼ tsp. garlic powder
¼ tsp. cumin
2 tsp. chopped parsley
1 Tbsp. lemon juice
1 tsp. salt

MIX all together and refrigerate for at least one hour.

Shredded lettuce
chopped cucumber
chopped tomatoes
chopped onion

PREPARE all vegetables and chill.

**6 small loaves Syrian bread
   (See page 102 for Mediter-
   ranean Pocket Bread)**
1 cup plain yogurt

CUT bread across center and open. Half fill with first mixture and top with chopped vegetables. Spoon yogurt on top. Sour cream or other dressing may be used instead. Lipton's onion soup mix may be mixed with yogurt or sour cream for a pleasing variation.

SERVES 6

EGYPTIAN STEW (Eggless)   158 Cal. per serving

2 Tbsp. oil
1 cup sliced onions
½ cup sliced green peppers

SAUTE vegetables in oil.

2 cups whole corn kernels
**2 cups cooked soybeans or
   limas**

ADD and cook on low heat for 15 minutes.

**1/3 cup tomatoes (fresh or
   canned)**
2 cups sliced zucchini squash
salt to taste

ADD and cook on low heat 15 to 20 minutes longer.

½ cup chopped parsley

ADD just before serving. In the Near East this is made with quite a lot of liquid and is served in bowls.

SERVES 8

BAKED BEANS HAWAIIAN STYLE   137 Cal. per serving

**4 cups cooked soy or navy
   beans**
**1 cup pineapple chunks or
   tidbits**

COMBINE and bake at 350* about 30 minutes or until juice of pineapple has cooked down.

SERVES 8

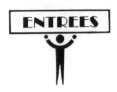

HUMMUS BI TAHINI (A distinctive dip) (Eggless)   27 Cal. per Tbsp.

1-20 oz. can garbanzos, drained
juice of 2 lemons
1 large onion, chopped
2 Tbsp. sesame tahini (ground, hulled sesame seeds)
1 minced garlic clove

COMBINE all ingredients in a blender. Let stand several hours for flavors to permeate. Serve with sesame seed crackers or Syrian bread.

YIELD: 2 cups

POLYNESIAN SOYAMEAT WITH PEACHES (Eggless)   184 Cal. per serving

3 cans 13 oz. chicken-style Soyameat
4 Tbsp. oil

CUT into thirds and brown in oil. Remove to another pot; reserve oil.

1 large onion
1 green pepper

QUARTER onion and separate into layers. Cut pepper in strips. Cook both in the oil until onion is transparent. Add to Soymeat.

1 - 29 oz. can sliced peaches

DRAIN and reserve liquid.

1 Tbsp. cornstarch
1 Tbsp. soy sauce
3 Tbsp. lemon juice

STIR into one cup of the reserved peach juice. Pour over soymeat and cook until clear and slightly thickened. Add peach slices.

2 medium tomatoes

CUT in sixths and add. Heat 5 minutes longer. Serve over hot rice.

SERVES 12

CURRIED RICE (Eggless)   256 Cal. per serving

1-10 oz. can mushroom soup
½ tsp. mild curry powder
½ medium onion, chopped

COMBINE soup, curry powder and onion; simmer slowly for 30 minutes.

3 cups cooked rice
¼ cup grated mild cheddar cheese
1-4 oz. can sliced mushrooms

ADD rice and pour into a 1½ quart casserole. Dot with cheese and mushrooms. Bake in a 350° oven for 15 minutes.

SERVES 4

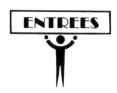
TOFU (Soy Cheese) FROM FLOUR

1 scant cup soy flour 1 quart water	BLEND together in liquifier till very smooth. Cook in double boiler for 20 minutes. Remove from heat.
3-4 Tbsp. lemon juice ¾ tsp. salt	ADD immediately. Stir once. Let cool. Do not disturb. In about 20 minutes the cheese will have formed a good curd. Strain in colander lined with a layer of cheese cloth. If very dry cheese is desired, place a weight on top. Can be made without salt for low salt diets. Then season with onion powder.

TOFU FROM DRY SOY BEANS

1 cup dry soy beans	SOAK overnight and discard water. Wash thoroughly. Liquify with about 3 cups water. Strain to remove skins and some fiber. Bring to a rolling boil.
juice of one lemon	ADD, stirring to form curds. Strain and chill.
salt to taste	

TOFU SERVING INSTRUCTIONS

1. Use in meatless dishes (See Tofu Loaf recipe).
2. Cube and add to stews and soups.
3. Scramble like eggs (see "Scrambled Eggs" recipe).
4. Cube and add to Chow Mein or Chop Suey.
5. Mix with mayonnaise, chopped sorrel and caraway or crushed dill seed for delicious sandwich filling.
6. Slice firm curd and bake in oven with tomato sauce or serve with gravy.

TOFU LOAF (Eggless)

1½ cup tofu
1 cup seasoned bread crumbs
   or 2 cups soft crumbled
   bread crumbs, seasoned
1½ cup white sauce
¼ tsp. salt or more
dash celery salt
¼ finely minced sauteed
   onion
	MIX well and pack into oiled baking dish. Place in a pan of water and bake at 375° for 50 minutes.

SERVES 6

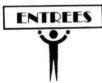

ENTREES

SCRAMBLED TOFU (Eggless)

3 Tbsp. oil
1 Tbsp. onion powder or ½ cup sauteed onion
1 Tbsp. soy sauce (or more)
½ tsp. salt (heaping)
¼ tsp. tumeric powder
¼ tsp. chicken style seasoning (optional)

STIR well in skillet.

2 cups homemade tofu (find also in Oriental food section of markets)

ADD to skillet and mix till seasonings are evenly distributed. Heat and serve like scrambled eggs. Good on buttered toast.

QUICK ONE-DISH ORIENTAL MEAL (Eggless)   150 Cal. per serving

6-8 gluten steaks*, cut in strips
bread crumbs or brewer's yeast
oil

BROWN steaks lighly in oil, after dipping in crumbs or yeast. Use electric fry pan if possible.

1-2 cups bean sprouts
1 cup chopped Chinese cabbage (Napa) or romaine lettuce
¼ cup green onions, sliced
¼ cup green peppers, sliced thin
1-4 oz. can mushrooms, drained

ADD vegetables in order given. (If making own sprouts, see page 117 for directions)

1 Tbsp. honey or brown sugar
2 Tbsp. soy sauce

ADD honey or sugar, and soy sauce. Cover and cook at low temperature for 10 minutes. Serve at once while vegetables are still crisp. Other vegetable combinations may be used. Serve in pan or dish in which it has been cooked. A chafing dish is nice. About 3-5 minutes before vegetables are done, lid may be removed and a handful of shredded spinach or other greens added. Serve with hot rice and a light dessert.

SERVES 6

QUICK CHOP SUEY (Eggless)   236 Cal. per serving

1 Tbsp. margarine or oil
¼ cup chopped onion
½ cup chopped celery

SAUTE onion and celery lightly in margarine.

1-5 oz. can water chestnuts
2 Tbsp. pimento
1-10-oz. can mushroom soup
1-13 oz. can Soyameat, chicken style
½ cup Soyameat liquid and water
2 Tbsp. soy sauce, or to taste

ADD remaining ingredients and heat until very hot. May be served over either rice or noodles.

SERVES 4

*See pg. 61

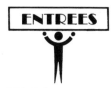

HOT CHINESE SALAD (Eggless)

266 Cal. per serving

1 lb. thin whole wheat
   spaghetti
1-10 oz. pkg. frozen broccoli
½ 10 oz. pkg. carrots
1 lb. fresh mushrooms

½ pkg. (4 oz.) frozen Soyameat, chicken style
1 tsp. salt
soy sauce

SERVES 8

COOK spaghetti; drain.

CHOP broccoli, cook and drain.
SLIVER carrots, cook and drain.
SLICE mushrooms, saute in margarine on high
heat; turn frequently.
DICE soyameat in small squares. Combine all in-
gredients.
ADD small amount of salt.
ADD to taste.

ORIENTAL SWEET 'N SOUR SAUCE (Eggless)

195 Cal. per serving

½ large green pepper,
   diced large
1 medium onion, diced large
2 stalks celery, slice diagonally
3 Tbsp. oil

SAUTE pepper, celery and onion in oil till clear.

4 Tbsp. lemon juice
1 cup pineapple juice
6 Tbsp. tomato puree
2 Tbsp. soy sauce
1 cup drained pineapple
   tidbits
2 Tbsp. brown sugar or to taste
¼ tsp. garlic salt

ADD and mix well.

1 Tbsp. cornstarch

MAKE smooth paste of cornstarch and a few drops
of cold water; add to mixture and cook till starch
is clear, stirring frequently.

1 cup Soyameat, chicken
   style, diced

ADD and heat through. Serve over rice.

SERVES 6

CHINESE NOODLE CASSEROLE (Eggless)

420 Cal. per serving

1 cup chopped celery
1 cup onion, chopped
1 8oz. can mushrooms
2 Tbsp. oil

MIX celery, onions and mushrooms and saute
in a little oil.

1-5 oz. can diced water
   chestnuts
1 5½ oz. can Chinese dry
   noodles
1-10 oz. can mushroom soup
1 cup liquid from mushrooms
   and water chestnuts
1¼ cups raw cashew nuts
2 pkgs. G. Washington's Broth

ADD rest of ingredients. Mix well and put in
greased casserole. Bake ½ hour at 350° or
until well-heated. If mixing the day before
baking, do not add noodles. Wait until ready to
bake, then add noodles. Mix well into mixture.

SERVES 6

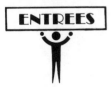

ENTREES

CHINESE STYLE SOYAMEAT (Eggless)

183 Cal. per serving

½ cup green onions
½ cup celery
½ cup string beans
½ cup finely cut carrots
4-oz. mushrooms
2 Tbsp. oil

CUT onions, celery and string beans on the diagonal. Saute all the vegetables in hot oil for 2 minutes.

1-13 oz. chicken-style
Soyameat

CUT soyameat in thin slices. Add with the gravy to the vegetables.

1-10 oz. can mushroom soup
1 tsp. chicken style seasoning

ADD and heat through.

2 tomatoes

CUT in 8 wedges and stir in. Remove from heat immediately and serve over hot rice, toast or noodles.

SERVES 6

VEGETABLE CURRY

286 Cal. per serving

1 onion, chopped
1-20 oz. can gluten cutlets*,
chopped
2 tsp. curry powder
2 tsp. salt
4 Tbsp. oil

SAUTE onion and gluten with curry.

5 cups whole milk
1 cup canned coconut milk,
(optional)
2 Tbsp. cornstarch
½ cup water

ADD milk and coconut milk to mixture. Dissolve cornstarch in water and add to gravy. Cook until slightly thickened.

4 medium sized potatoes,
diced
3 carrots, diced
1-10 oz. pkg. frozen green
beans
2 tsp. salt

COOK vegetables in water. When tender, drain and add to curry sauce.

4 hard boiled eggs

SLICE eggs and stir into curry. Serve over rice with sliced bananas, flaked coconut, raisins and peanuts as garnishes.

SERVES 10

NOODLES ROMANOFF (Eggless)

281 Cal. per serving

3 cups cooked noodles
1 cup cottage cheese
½ cup sliced almonds
1 cup sour cream
½ onion, minced
1 Tbsp. soy sauce
½ tsp. salt
¼ cup crumbs or wheat germ

MIX all ingredients together. Bake in 2 quart baking dish. Sprinkle buttered bread crumbs or wheat germ on top. Bake at 350° for 40 minutes.

SERVES 6

*See pg. 61

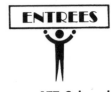
RUNZA

177 Cal. each

1½ cups milk, scalded ¼ cup corn oil ½ cup sugar 1 tsp. salt	COMBINE milk, oil, sugar and salt. Cool to luke-warm.
1 pkg. yeast	ADD yeast and stir well.
2 eggs, well beaten	ADD eggs and mix.
4½ cups flour	ADD flour and mix to smooth, soft dough. Turn out on floured surface and knead lightly. Place dough in greased mixing bowl. Cover and let rise till double in bulk.
1-20 oz. can meatless burger* 1 large head cabbage, shredded 2 medium onions, chopped 2 cloves garlic, minced 1 tsp. salt 1 Tbsp. mushroom powder (optional) 1 tsp. sage	BRAISE cabbage, onions, and garlic in oil. Add burger and seasonings. Cover and steam for 10 minutes.
YIELD: 20	Place dough on floured surface and roll into a square ¼ inch thick. Cut in 6 inch squares. Place ¾ cup filling in center of each square. Bring corners of square to center and pinch edges together firmly. Brush each square with oil. Bake at 400° for 15 minutes or until a golden brown. Serve with margarine or mushroom gravy while warm.

CONTINENTAL STROGANOFF (Eggless)

177 Cal. per serving

1-20 oz. can meatless steaks* 1 - 4 oz. can mushrooms 2 Tbsp. margarine	DRAIN vegetable steaks and mushrooms, reserving liquid. Cut steaks in strips. Brown in margarine.
1 envelope Lipton's dry onion soup mix 3 Tbsp. flour 1 cup milk ½ cup sour cream or Soyamel Sour Kreem (page 119)	ADD soup mix and flour; gradually stir in milk and reserved liquid to blend. Add sour cream; heat. Serve over rice.

SERVES 8

*See pg. 61

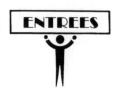

VARENIKU (Russian Cheese Pockets)   219 Cal. per serving

FILLING:

1 lb. dry cottage cheese
1 egg
¼ tsp. salt
1 Tbsp. wheat germ
1 Tbsp. cream cheese

MIX together in a pan and press down so it will be easy to work with.

DOUGH:

2½ cups sifted white flour
¼ tsp. salt
1 egg
½ cup milk or water
1 Tbsp. oil

BREAK egg into small bowl and beat. Add oil and milk. Sift flour and salt together. Add to egg mixture and knead well. If dough is too soft, add more flour. Roll out dough ⅛ inch thick on floured board and cut with a 3 inch cookie cutter. Place 1 Tbsp. full of cheese filling into each circle of dough. Fold over and pinch together like an apple turnover. Drop filled dough pieces into large kettle of boiling water and cook about 2 minutes. Drain in colander with small amount of butter so they won't stick together. Place in baking dish and cover with sour cream or sweet cream. Bake 350° for 30 min.

SERVES 8

HUNGARIAN EGG BARLEY GOULASH (Eggless)   315 Cal. per serving

4 large onions
4 cups Goodman's egg barley
½ cup olive oil

SLICE onions and simmer with the egg barley in oil until golden yellow.

1 tsp. paprika
½ tsp. salt

ADD and cover immediately with water. Add more salt to taste, if desired. Cook until barley is half done.

5 medium potatoes
2 peppers, chopped

PEEL and dice potatoes and add when barley is half done. Add hot water as needed. Cook covered, stirring frequently. When done it should be thick enough so that the spoon will stand up in the mixture.

SERVES 8

The Egg and I . . .

Pros . . .

- Eggs are the source of protein of highest biological value
- Used as a protein standard in nutritional research
- Good source of riboflavin (Vitamin B_2), Vitamins A and D
- Good source of iron (in yolk)
- Supplies phosphorous and copper
- Noted for eight specific cooking qualities, including binding, coating, jelling and clarifying

Cons . . .

- Yolk has highest single source of cholestrol
- Disease in chickens increasing
  - Lymphomatosis, a cancer virus transmitted through eggs, (although no evidence of transmission to man). Can be destroyed by thorough heating. [1]
  - Cracked eggs carry a high incidence of infectious bacteria, especially Salmonella, and should not be used [2]
- Allergenic for some people

Egg Substitutes . . .

- 2 egg whites for 1 whole egg
- "Binders" to replace egg in some recipes: soy flour, cornstarch or thick white sauce
- Eggbeaters (Fleischmann, 625 Madison Ave., New York, N. Y. 10022)
    yolks removed and replaced with polyunsaturated fat
- Jolly Joan Egg Extender (Ener-g-Food, Inc., Seattle, Washington, 98134)
- Eggstra (Tillie Lewis Foods, Inc., Stockton, Calif. 95201)
    80% yolk removed and replaced by polyunsaturated fat

WARNING!!

"Americans should be encouraged to modify habits with regard to all five major sources of fat in the U. S. diet — meats, dairy products, baked goods, eggs, table and cooking fats — [3]

Three important FAT definitions . . .

- SATURATED fats are usually solid at room temperature, and in the diet tend to raise the serum cholesterol (e.g. butter)
- MONOUNSATURATED fats are liquid at room temperature, (e.g. olive oil) and have a neutral effect on serum cholesterol
- POLYUNSATURATED fats are liquid oils which tend to lower the serum cholesterol (e.g. corn oil)

What is hydrogenation?

- Unsaturated vegetable oils are reacted with hydrogen under pressure
- The vegetable oil becomes SATURATED with hydrogen and a solid fat is produced
- This improves the shelf life or may give a more suitable solid consistency
- BUT — the beneficial polyunsaturated feature with its serum cholesterol lowering ability is now lost in direct proportion to degree of hydrogenation

Dietary fat – serum cholesterol – heart attacks

- As dietary fat increases, serum cholesterol and heart attack rates also rise
- Heart attack risk in men aged 40-59 is 4 times greater with serum cholesterol above 260 mg/dl than those with level under 200
- Heart attack risk is 4 times greater if triglyceride level is above 250 compared with under 150
- Heart attack rates are low until the dietary fat is 30-40% of the TOTAL CALORIES
- The average American diet has 40% or MORE of its calories in fat which should definitely be lowered
- There are approximately ONE MILLION heart attacks each year in the United States
- Less than 10% of total calories should be from SATURATED FATS (see pg. 30 also)

References:
1. Lymphomatosis in Chickens, Circular #970, U.S.D.A. 1959
2. J. Amer. Med. Asso., May 15, 1954, p. 300
3. Primary Prevention of the Atherosclerotic Diseases, Circulation, Vol. 42, 1972, pg. 34
4. Inter-Society Commission for Heart Disease Resources, New York, N. Y. 1970

Eggless (LEGUMES — NUTS — GRAINS)

BASIC LOAF RECIPE FOR LEGUMES

1 cup legumes, cooked
1 cup bread crumbs, wheat germ or ground nuts
1 cup liquid — milk, tomato juice, etc.
seasonings to taste — garlic, onions, etc.

SERVES 6

MIX all ingredients thoroughly. Bake in loaf pan in 350° oven until firm, about 30 minutes.

CASHEW LOAF

325 Cal. per serving

2 cups raw cashews
2 cups soy or evaporated milk
2 large onions
4 slices whole wheat bread

2 Tbsp. soy sauce
1 tsp. salt
2 Tbsp. dried parsley
½ tsp. celery seed

SERVES 8

BLEND all in blender or put through food grinder, all except the milk. If you grind the ingredients, pour milk over the top.

ADD and mix well. Place in well greased baking pan and bake at 350° until firm, about 40 minutes.

PECAN LOAF

282 Cal. per serving

1 cup pecans
1 cup dry bread crumbs

1 small onion
2 medium sized potatoes
1½ cups milk

½ cup soy flour
1 tsp. salt
½ tsp. sage

SERVES 6

GRIND nuts and crackers separately in blender.

CHOP onion and potatoes in milk in the blender. Add to nut mixture.

ADD and mix well. Pour into greased loaf pan. Dot the top with small pea-sized pieces of margarine. Bake at 350° for 30 minutes. Serve with brown gravy.

SUNFLOWER LOAF

279 Cal. per serving

½ cup ground sunflower seeds
½ cup bread crumbs
1 cup ground walnuts
½ cup grated raw potato
1 tsp. salt
1 cup milk, soy or dairy
3 Tbsp. grated onion
1 Tbsp. oil

SERVES 6

MIX all ingredients well. Let stand covered for ½ hour. Bake at 350° for one hour.

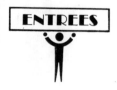

ENTREES

LENTIL LOAF
208 Cal. per serving

1 ½ cups lentils, cooked	MASH.
2 stalks celery, chopped ½ medium onion, chopped 2 Tbsp. oil	SAUTE in oil and add to lentils.
1 cup dry bread crumbs ½ cup crushed potato chips ½ tsp. sage 1 tsp. poultry seasoning 1 tsp. Bakon yeast ½ tsp. oregano ½ cup evaporated milk	ADD to above ingredients. Mix and bake in greased loaf pan for one hour at 350°.

SERVES 6

RICE NUT LOAF
346 Cal. per serving

1 cup peanut butter 1 cup water	CREAM together until smooth.
2 cups cooked brown rice 2 Tbsp. finely chopped onion 1 tsp. sage salt to taste	ADD to peanut butter. The mixture will be quite thin. Pour into a small greased casserole. Bake at 350° for one hour.
1 10 oz. can tomato soup	HEAT undiluted soup and pour over as a sauce.

SERVES 6

CASHEW NUT CASSEROLE
235 Cal. per serving

1 cup cashew nuts, chopped *Rinsed*	MIX all together. Bake 1 hour at 350°.
1 cup onions, chopped	
1 cup mushrooms, chopped	
1 cup celery, chopped -	¼ tsp salt .
2 Tbsp. oil	
~~1 cup dry egg noodles (fine)~~	
~~1 tsp. Accent~~	
2 cup dry Chinese noodles	
~~1 tsp. Accent~~	
1 cup liquid from mushrooms (add water to make one cup if not enough liquid)	
½ tsp. salt	

SERVES 6 *Can Mushroom Soup*

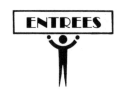

CARROT RICE LOAF

291 Cal. per serving

½ cup peanut butter
1 cup milk, soy or dairy

CREAM together until smooth.

1 small onion, grated
3 Tbsp. oil

SIMMER until onion is soft, but not brown.

½ tsp. salt
⅛ tsp. sage
½ cup whole wheat bread crumbs

ADD to the onion mixture.

2 cups grated carrots
1 cup cooked brown rice

COMBINE and then add all ingredients, mixing thoroughly. Bake in a greased pan at 350° about one hour.

SERVES 6

SOYBEAN CARROT LOAF

272 Cal. per serving

4 cups cooked mashed soybeans
2 cups shredded carrots
1 chopped onion
½ cup chopped celery
1 cup bread crumbs, dry
1 cup wheat germ
2 tsp. salt
¼ cup melted margarine (optional)

MIX all ingredients thoroughly. Pack into a well greased pan. Bake at 350° about 45 minutes.

SERVES 8

WALNUT STUFFING BALLS

405 Cal. per serving

4 cups bread crumbs
1 cup chopped walnuts
1 tsp. salt
½ tsp. sage
½ tsp. thyme
½ tsp. basil
½ cup diced celery
½ cup chopped parsley

TOSS all dry ingredients together.

1 chopped onion
½ cup oil

SAUTE onion in oil and add to crumb mixture.

2 vegetable bouillon cubes
1 cup boiling water

DISSOLVE cubes in water. You may use 2 tsp. McKay's chicken style seasoning instead of cubes. Add just enough of the bouillon to moisten the mixture. Shape into 2 inch balls. Place on oiled baking sheet. Bake at 375° about 20 minutes until crisp and brown.

SERVES 8

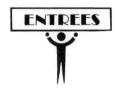

ENTREES

CHICK PEA CASSEROLE

250 Cal. per serving

4 cups cooked chick peas
¼ cup water or vegetable
  broth
1 can mushroom soup
3 Tbsp. parsley, chopped
other seasonings as desired
1 tsp. soy sauce

COMBINE all ingredients. Bake covered at 350°
for 45 minutes.

SERVES 6

SOY SOUFFLE

176 Cal. per serving

1 cup dry soybeans

SOAK overnight. Liquify in blender with about 2
cups water. This should make 5 cups pulp.

2 Tbsp. oil
2 tsp. chicken-style seasoning
¼ tsp. Italian seasoning
1½ tsp. salt
1 tsp. Accent

ADD and mix well. Pour into a shallow pan so
that souffle is not more than two inches thick.
Bake at 300° for 1½ to 2 hours. This will puff
up but shrink down as it cools. Serve with tartar
sauce as with fish.

SERVES 6

NUT POTATO PATTIES

239 Cal. per serving

½ cup ground nuts
1 cup mashed potatoes
½ tsp salt
1 Tbsp. brewer's yeast

MIX together.

1 cup boiling water
½ cup oatmeal, dry

STIR oats into water and cook until thick. Add
to above and mix.

½ cup whole wheat flour
¼ cup brewer's yeast

MIX for a breading meal. Dip patties into this
mixture and fry until golden brown.

SERVES 4

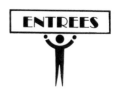

CASHEW-PIMIENTO "CHEESE"

256 Cal. per ½ cup serving

½ cup raw cashews
1 cup water

BLEND water and cashews.

½ tsp. salt
2 tsp. onion powder
2 Tbsp. soy "milk" powder
   (optional)
3-4 Tbsp. brewer's yeast

ADD to blended mixture.

1 cup oil

ADD oil to blender very slowly to thicken.

¼ cup lemon juice
2-3 pimentos

ADD to blender and blend for a short time. Use on bread or in recipes below.

YIELD: 3 cups

GREEN RICE

204 Cal. per serving

2 cups cooked rice
1 cup grated American cheese
   or ½ cup Cashew-Pimento
   "Cheese"
1 cup chopped parsley
¼ cup oil (2 Tbsp. if using
   Cashew-Pimento "Cheese"
2 cups evaporated milk
1 onion, grated
1 clove garlic
1 tsp. salt

MIX cheese with hot rice. Add other ingredients in order given. Bake in oiled casserole for 45 minutes at 350°.

SERVES 8

CAULIFLOWER DELIGHT

121 Cal. per serving

1 - 8 oz. can mushrooms
¼ cup green pepper, diced
1/3 cup margarine
¼ cup flour
2 cups milk
1 tsp. salt
6 oz. pimento cheese or ¼
   cup cashew "cheese"
   (above)

BROWN mushrooms and green pepper in margarine. Blend in flour. Stir in milk; cook until thick, stirring constantly. Add salt. Grate pimento cheese. Stir into sauce.

1 medium head cauliflower

BREAK cauliflower into medium size pieces. Cook for 10 minutes. In a greased casserole, place half of the cauliflower and cover with half of the sauce; repeat. Bake 350° for 15 minutes.

SERVES 8

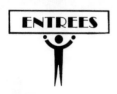

ENTREES

LENTIL POTATO PATTIES

260 Cal. per serving

1 chopped onion
4 Tbsp. oil
½ tsp. sage

COMBINE in pan and simmer a few minutes to soften the onion, but do not brown.

2 cups cooked lentils
2 cups mashed potatoes
½ cup chopped pecans
salt to taste

ADD and mix well. Form into small patties and place on an oiled cookie sheet. Brush top with oil and bake at 400° until brown, about 15—20 minutes. Serve with gravy or tomato sauce.

SERVES 6

QUICK LENTIL PATTIES

248 Cal. per serving

1 small onion, chopped
2 Tbsp. oil

SAUTE onion in oil.

2 cups cooked mashed lentils
½ cup chopped walnuts
1 tsp. salt

MIX all ingredients. Form into patties. Place on an oiled cookie sheet and brown in oven. Serve with gravy or tomato sauce.

SERVES 4

SOY CUTLETS

173 Cal. per serving

½ cup dry soybeans

COVER with water and soak overnight.

1 cup water

DRAIN soy beans and whiz in blender with water until fine, or grind fine and add water.

or walnuts
½ cup pecan meal
1 cup oatmeal, dry
1 medium onion, chopped
½ cup celery, chopped
~~½ tsp. salt~~
3 Tbsp. soy sauce

ADD remaining ingredients and mix well. Let stand about 10 minutes to absorb moisture. Drop by tablespoons on lightly oiled skillet. Brown lightly on both sides. Place in baking dish. Bake 20 minutes at 350°. Cover with your favorite tomato sauce or brown gravy and bake until heated through.

SERVES 6

Add _ Meat Tenderizer unseasoned

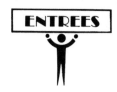

WHEAT GERM OATMEAL BURGERS

260 Cal. per serving

1 **medium chopped onion** 2 **Tbsp. oil**	SAUTE onion in oil until yellow.

1 ½ **cups oatmeal, dry**
1 **cup wheat germ**
1 **tsp. salt**
2 **Tbsp. soy sauce**
½ **tsp. sage**
½ **tsp. garlic salt**
½ **cup chopped nuts**
13 **oz. can evaporated milk**

COMBINE all these ingredients with the onion and let stand while making the following sauce.

2 **Tbsp. flour**
2 **Tbsp. margarine**
½ **cup milk**

BLEND together and cook until thick. Add to the rest of the ingredients. Mix well. Drop by tablespoons into hot oil. Brown on both sides. Serve with your favorite gravy.

SERVES 8

PECAN PATTIES

233 Cal. per serving

1 **cup chopped pecans**
1 **cup cooked brown rice**
1 **cup soy or dairy milk**
1 **Tbsp. soy flour**
1 **tsp. salt**
1 **Tbsp. dry parsley flakes**
½ **cup bread crumbs**
½ **cup wheat germ**
1 **Tbsp. dry minced onion**
dash of garlic powder
   (optional)

COMBINE all ingredients. Shape into patties. Place on an oiled cookie sheet. Brush top with oil. Bake at 350° until brown, about 30 minutes.

SERVE with gravy or tomato sauce.

SERVES 6

NUT MEAT BALLS

233 Cal. per serving

1 **cup cooked millet, wheat**
   or rice
½ **cup finely ground pecans**
¼ **cup finely ground sun-**
   flower seeds
1 **Tbsp. finely ground cashew**
   nuts
½ **cup wheat germ**
1 **tsp. salt**
½ **tsp. Italian seasoning**

COMBINE all ingredients, mixing well. Roll into balls. Sprinkle with paprika. Bake on oiled cookie sheet 30 minutes at 325°.

SERVE with gravy or tomato sauce.

SERVES 4

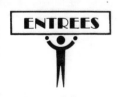

ENTREES

50% oil
50% lethicin

VEGETABLE BURGERS

243 Cal. per serving

1 medium potato
1 small onion
½ cup walnuts or pecans

GRIND or chop in blender.

4 Tbsp. oil

SAUTE in oil ground mixture until soft.

1 cup cooked oatmeal
1 cup bread crumbs
1 tsp. salt
½ tsp. sage
2 Tbsp. soy sauce

ADD remaining ingredients. Mix thoroughly. Form into burger patties and fry until brown on both sides, or bake on oiled sheet in 350° oven till brown.

40 min

SERVES 6

SPROUTED WHEAT BURGERS

2 cups sprouted wheat
2 cups steamed barley
2 Tbsp. peanut butter
2 Tbsp. oil
2 Tbsp. soy sauce
1 Tbsp. onion powder or ¼
  cup raw onion
½ tsp. salt
½ tsp. sage
½ cup whole wheat bread
  crumbs

MIX all ingredients together and brown quickly in a skillet on both sides. Place between burger buns and serve with health catsup. May also be served with gravy as a meatless main dish.

SERVES 8

OAT-NUT BURGERS

290 Cal. per serving

2 cups oatmeal, dry
1 cup pecan meal
1½ tsp. salt
½ tsp. Italian seasoning
13 oz. can evaporated milk

COMBINE and let stand one hour, or less if you are in a hurry. Garlic powder or other favorite seasonings may be added.

1 medium minced onion
1 cup chopped celery
2 Tbsp. oil

SAUTE onion and celery in oil. Add to first mixture. Form into small patties. Fry over medium heat until browned on both sides. Place in baking dish. Bake at 375° for 20 minutes.

1 10 oz. can mushroom soup
  diluted

COVER with soup or your favorite gravy. Bake at 375° for 10 minutes more.

SERVES 8

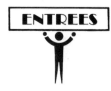

ENTREES

ECONOMY BURGERS

282 Cal. per serving

2½ cups water
5 Tbsp. soy sauce
¼ cup oil
1 clove minced garlic
1 medium onion, chopped
¼ tsp. Italian seasoning
1 Tbsp. Bakon yeast, optional

BOIL. Remove from heat.

2 cups oatmeal, dry
1 cup finely chopped nuts

MIX oats and nuts together, then sprinkle gradually into boiling broth. Let stand until most of liquid is absorbed. Then stir lightly until just mixed. Drop by spoonfuls on oiled cookie sheet. Press flat. Bake at 350° about 30 minutes.

SERVES 6

EGGPLANT PATTIES

207 Cal. per serving

1 eggplant, diced

COOK eggplant in salted water until soft, drain and mash.

½ cup wheat germ
½ cup ground walnuts
½ cup herb seasoned crumbs
½ cup oatmeal, dry
½ tsp. Accent
½ tsp. garlic powder

MIX eggplant with crumbs and oatmeal.
Allow to stand to absorb moisture. Add seasoning. Fry in oil until brown. Serve with brown gravy or tomato sauce.

SERVES 4

CASHEW PIMENTO "CHEESE" MACARONI

329 Cal. per serving

2 cups macaroni

COOK according to directions and drain.

1-1/3 cups water
1 cup raw cashews
1 tsp. salt

WHIZ in blender.

½ cup oil

ADD oil slowly while continuing to blend.

1/3 cup lemon juice
4 oz. jar pimientos
1 tsp. onion powder
1 tsp. garlic salt
3 Tbsp. brewer's yeast

ADD and blend till smooth.

1 medium chopped onion
2 Tbsp. oil

SAUTE onion and mix with macaroni. Place in baking dish. Pour the sauce over the macaroni. Bake at 350° for 45 minutes. Top with bread crumbs or wheat germ if desired, before baking.

SERVES 8

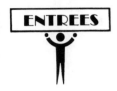

CREAM CHEESE BALLS

354 Cal. per serving

4 Tbsp. margarine
4 Tbsp. flour
1 cup milk

COOK to make thick cream sauce from margarine, flour and milk.

½ cup wheat germ
8 oz. cream cheese
1 cup chopped nuts
½ cup cracker crumbs
1 pkg. Lipton's onion soup

ADD remaining ingredients and mix well. Roll into small balls. Roll in additional cracker crumbs. or breading meal. Fry until golden brown (deep fat frying is ideal, but not necessary). Serve as is or with sauce of choice.

SERVES 8

JEWISH VEGETARIAN "CHOPPED LIVER"

17 Cal. per Tbsp.

1 cup cooked lentils
½ cup pecans
1-10 oz. pkg. frozen string beans, cooked
2 large onions, sauted in oil

GRIND all ingredients.   A hard boiled egg may be ground in also.

1 Tbsp. soy sauce
1 tsp. chicken-style seasoning
garlic salt to taste

ADD seasonings. Mix well and refrigerate to blend in flavors. Serve on crackers as hors d'oeuvres.

YIELD: 4 CUPS

LENTIL POTTAGE

301 Cal. per serving

1 cup lentils, dry
¾ cups brown rice, dry
1 Tbsp. salt
7 cups water

COMBINE in sauce pan. Cook covered about 30 minutes.

4 onions
½ cup olive oil

SLICE onions and saute in oil until lightly browned. Add to lentils and rice. Cook all uncovered over low flame for 15 minutes, or until most of liquid is absorbed. Delicious hot or cold.

SERVES 8

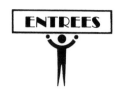

STUFFED CABBAGE ENTREE

258 Cal. per serving

10 green cabbage leaves

STEAM for 5 minutes.

2 cups cooked brown rice
1 cup chopped walnuts
½ cup diced onion
½ cup diced celery
½ cup chopped spinach
½ tsp. salt
2 Tbsp. soy sauce

MIX well. Fill each leaf with a heaping table-spoon of mixture and roll into a neat roll. Tuck ends under so mixture will not spill while baking. Lightly oil baking dish. Put any leftover mixture on bottom of dish. Place cabbage rolls on top, close together. Cover and bake at 350° for 25 minutes. Serve with tomato sauce.

SERVES 5

BARLEY PILAF

242 Cal. per serving

4 Tbsp. margarine
2 medium onions, chopped
1 cup fresh mushrooms or
   4 oz. can drained

SAUTE lightly the vegetables in the margarine. Then lift out from margarine and place in casserole.

2 cups barley

BROWN barley in same skillet, stirring constantly. Add to casserole and mix.

4 cups hot water
4 pkgs. G. Washington broth

COMBINE to make broth and pour over casserole. You may use 4 tsp. McKay's Chicken-Style seasoning for the broth. Cover and bake at 350° for one hour.

SERVES 8

HOLIDAY PILAF

200 Cal. per serving

1 cup diced celery
1 small onion, chopped
4 Tbsp. oil

SIMMER together 5 minutes

2 vegetable bouillon cubes
½ tsp. salt
4 oz. sliced mushrooms
   with liquid
8 ripe olives, sliced
2 Tbsp. raisins

ADD and bring to a boil.

1 cup cooked peas
2 cups cooked brown rice

ADD and heat through. Toss lightly with a fork. Serve immediately.

SERVES 4

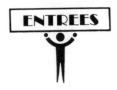

PECAN TOMATO ROAST

318 Cal. per serving

2 cups pecans, chopped
1 cup cooked potatoes,
   chopped in small pieces
1 cup celery
1 small onion, sauted
1-4 oz. can tomato sauce
1 cup bread crumbs
2 tsp. soy sauce or seasoned
   salt to taste

MIX all together. Place in greased casserole and
bake for 45 minutes at 350° For variation, 1
4 oz. can mushrooms, chopped, may be added.

SERVES 8

WALNUT BALLS

237 Cal. per serving

1 cup ground raw potatoes
1 cup dry whole wheat bread
   crumbs (ground)
2 tsp. soy flour
3 chopped onions
1 cup ground walnuts
½ tsp. sage
½ tsp. salt

MIX thoroughly. Form into balls. Put in baking
dish. Pour your favorite gravy over them and
bake 20-30 minutes at 375°.

SERVES 6

LENTIL TOMATO LOAF

303 Cal. per serving

¾ cup chopped onion
4 Tbsp. oil
1 tsp. soy sauce

BRAISE onion in oil and soy sauce.

3 Tbsp. flour

STIR in flour and cook a few minutes.

¾ cup tomato juice

ADD slowly stirring constantly.

1½ cups cooked lentils
¾ cup cereal flakes
¾ cup chopped walnuts
1 tsp. salt

MASH lentils. Add with rest of ingredients to
the onion tomato mixture. Turn into well-greased
loaf pan. Bake at 375° about 45 minutes.

SERVES 6

COTTAGE CHEESE ROAST

303 Cal. per serving

1 medium chopped onion
3 Tbsp. margarine

SIMMER onion in margarine until golden.

2 cups cottage cheese
2 cups whole wheat bread
   crumbs, dry
½ cup ground nuts
1 tsp. sage
1 tsp. salt

MIX thoroughly and combine with onion. Put in
flat baking pan and bake at 350° until brown,
about 40 minutes.

SERVES 6

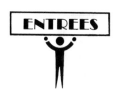
MAKE YOUR OWN GLUTEN (WHEAT PROTEIN)

8 cups bread flour
2½-3 cups water

MIX flour with enough water to make a stiff dough. Form dough into a ball and knead about 10 minutes. Place in bowl and cover with additional water. Let stand 30 minutes or overnight. Knead dough with hands underwater to wash out the starch. Pour off the starchy water and cover with more water. Continue washing until water is almost clear. You now have the concentrated protein and you may use it in the following ways.

STEAKS FROM HOMEMADE GLUTEN

4 cups vegetable water
3 Tbsp. oil
2 cups chopped onion
6 Tbsp. soy sauce
½ cup tomato juice
1 tsp. salt

COMBINE all ingredients and bring to a boil. Adjust seasoning to make a savory broth to your taste. Slice gluten made from the above recipe into steaks. Simmer in boiling broth for 15 minutes, then boil, covered for 30 minutes. Keep steaks in the liquid until ready to use. Cool and refrigerate. They may be breaded and fried when ready to use.

GLUTEN PUFFS

Tear off walnut sized pieces of homemade gluten. Place on a baking sheet and bake at 350° until the balls puff up and are light. Then drop into the savory broth and proceed as above. As an alternate, the pieces may be deep fat fried instead of baking. They will be puffed up and light.

---

* MEATLESS BURGER:

Any of the following may be used in recipes calling for meatless burger: Glutenburger (above), Vegetarian Burger (Worthington); Choplet Burger (Worthington); Vegeburger (Loma Linda); Granburger (Worthington) after dehydration. 1 20 oz. can = 2-1/3 cups.

* MEATLESS STEAKS: Cutlets, Choplets (Worthington); Tender Bits and Dinner Cuts (Loma Linda); Gluten Steaks (see above)

Gravies and Sauces

DELICIOUS BROWN GRAVY

1 small onion 4 Tbsp. oil	DICE onion. Saute in oil.
½ cup chopped cashews or almonds	ADD nuts. Brown for 5 minutes.
3 rounded Tbsp. flour	STIR in flour and brown lightly.
3 cups cold potato water more liquid if necessary Vegex or soy sauce to taste	STIR in 2 cups cold liquid. Have other liquid ready, hot if desired. This liquid can be any kind of vegetable stock, mushroom liquid or all potato water can be used. Plain water will not give the same flavor. When flour mixture begins to thicken in pan, add the additional liquid and stir as it thickens. This should not be a very thick mixture. Season with Vegex or soy sauce then salt to taste.

MUSHROOM GRAVY

1 small onion, diced 1 - 4 oz. can mushrooms 1 can mushroom soup soy sauce to taste	DRAIN mushrooms, reserving the liquid. Saute onion and mushrooms in margarine. Add mushroom soup, soy sauce, and liquid from mushrooms to reach desired consistency.

CASHEW NUT GRAVY

1 cup water ½ cup raw cashews	WHIZ in blender at least 2 minutes. You must use raw cashews as it is the starch that thickens.
2 tsp. Bakon yeast 1 tsp. Italian seasoning 1 Tbsp. soy sauce 1 pkg. G. Washington Broth	ADD seasonings. Other favorite seasonings may be used as desired. Try 1 Tbsp. McKay's Chicken Style Seasoning and 2 Tbsp. Bakon yeast. Pour into skillet.
¾ cup water	DILUTE with water and bring to a boil. Stir constantly until thickened.

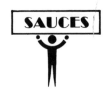

WHITE SAUCE

THIN	MEDIUM	THICK	BLEND well over medium heat.
1 Tbsp. oil	2 Tbsp. oil	3 Tbsp. oil	
1 Tbsp. flour	2 Tbsp. flour	4 Tbsp. flour	
¼ tsp. salt	¼ tsp. salt	¼ tsp. salt	
1 cup cold milk	1 cup cold milk	1 cup cold milk	STIR in gradually. Bring to a boil. Cook 2 minutes.

ALMOND CREAM SAUCE

Follow recipe for medium white sauce adding 1/3 cup blanched sliced almonds.

PARSLEY CREAM SAUCE

Follow recipe for medium cream sauce adding ¼ cup minced parsley.

CHEESE SAUCE

Follow recipe for medium white sauce adding ½ cup greated American cheese. Stir until melted.

MUSHROOM CREAM SAUCE

Follow recipe for medium white sauce adding 1 cup sauteed mushrooms and ½ tsp. onion powder. If you use canned mushrooms use part of the liquid with the milk.

CARROT TARTAR SAUCE

¾ cup water
½ cup cooked potato
¼ cup cooked carrots
1 Tbsp. oil
¼ tsp. salt
¼ tsp. Accent
1 Tbsp. lemon juice

LIQUIFY in blender until smooth. You may also add a small amount of smoked flavoring such as ¼ tsp. Smokene or Bakon yeast if desired. Serve to top leaves, patties or vegetables. After pouring on a leaf or eggplant, you may bake a few minutes more until set and bubbly.

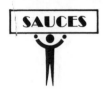

SAUCES

MUSHROOM SAUCE

1 small chopped onion 1 stalk chopped celery 2 Tbsp. margarine	SAUTE lightly.
½ pound sliced mushrooms	ADD and cook 5 minutes.
½ tsp. salt ½ tsp. basil 1 Tbsp. flour	SPRINKLE in and mix.
1 cup water 1 Tbsp. lemon juice, optional	ADD and cook until sauce bubbles and thickens. Maks about 2 cups.

CHILI SAUCE

4 cups tomato pulp 2 minced onions 4 green peppers, bell 2 red peppers, bell ¼ tsp. salt ½ Tbsp. celery salt	COOK, stirring often to prevent sticking. Cook slowly, boiling down to about ½ original bulk.
4 Tbsp. honey 2 Tbsp. lemon juice	SWEETEN and sour to taste with honey and lemon juice. Can in hot jars.

LEMON JUICE KETCHUP

1 - 6 oz. can tomato paste 2 Tbsp. oil 2 tsp. honey 1 tsp. salt 2 Tbsp. lemon juice onion and garlic powder to taste	MIX well and refrigerate to blend flavors. This has no preservatives so must be kept in refrigerator.

TARTAR SAUCE

1 cup soy mayonnaise 1 Tbsp. lemon dill pickles 1 Tbsp. flaked parsley 1 small onion, minced 2 Tbsp. pimento, chopped 2 Tbsp. soy sauce	MIX all ingredients and store in refrigerator until used. Storage improves the flavor.

ITALIAN TOMATO SAUCE — See page 32

SPANISH TOMATO SAUCE — See page 32

Versatile Vegetables . . .

Did you know that some vegetables can be served in the menu from "soup to seed"? Take the lowly squash . . .

- Squash Soup (pg. 80)
- Zucchini Patties (pg. 68)
- Golden Raisin-Nut Squash Bread (pg. 99)
- Zesty Zucchini Salad (pg. 123)
- Honey Baked Acorn Squash (pg. 70)
- Eggless Squash Pie (pg. 144)
- Buttered, salted pumpkin seed

Notable winter squash properties . . .

- 8,610 International units Vitamin A/cup[1]
- 130 calories/cup
- High in Niacin, Riboflavin and Thiamine
- Good amounts of calcium and phosphorus
- Good potassium content; very little sodium
- 4 Grams protein/cup
- 27 mg. ascorbic acid (Vitamin C)/cup
- Negligible fat

Other versatile vegetables . . .

- Tomatoes: soup, salad, vegetable, sauces, bread, dessert
- Carrots: soup, salad, entree, vegetable, bread, dessert
- Potatoes: soup, salad, vegetable, entree, bread

.S. But are tomatoes and squash really vegetables? (See pg. 118)

Nutritional Nuggets . . .

One day sample menu Vegetarian-milk-egg diet

- **Breakfast**

	gms. protein	Calories[2]
Orange Juice (1 cup)	2	110
Cooked oatmeal (1 cup)	5	130
Raisins (½ oz.)	0	40
Toast, whole wheat	3	65
Margarine (1 tsp.)	0	35
Whole milk (½ cup)	4	80
	14	460

Total:

58 gms. protein

1375 calories

- **Dinner**

Special K Loaf	15	230
Baked potato	3	90
Margarine (2 tsp.)	0	70
Broccoli (1 cup)	5	40
Carrot sticks (1 carrot)	1	20
Whole milk (1 cup)	8	160
	32	610

Note that this
menu is low
in calories
yet the
**PROTEIN INTAKE
IS MORE THAN
THE DAILY
ALLOWANCE**

- **Supper**

Lentils (½ cup)	7	90
Bread, whole wheat	3	65
Cole Slaw (1 cup)	1	80
Apple	1	70
	12	305

Do Athletes need MEAT for strength?

- On a fat and protein (meat) diet athletes' maximum endurance on strenuous exercise was 57 minutes
- On a normal mixed diet (meat and vegetables) maximum work time by athletes was 114 minutes.
- A high carbohydrate MEATLESS diet gave endurance of 167 minutes [3]

References:
1. Nutrition Value of Foods, U. S. Dept. of Agriculture, Bulletin #72
2. Nutrition Value of Foods, U. S. Dept. of Agriculture, Bulletin #72.
3. Astrand, Per-Olaf, Something Old and Something New . . . Very New, Nutrition Today, June 1968, pp. 9-11

Vegetables

HERBED GREEN BEANS

68 Cal. per serving

1 pound green beans

WASH, remove ends, and cut crosswise into thin diagonal slices. Cook, covered in one half inch of boiling water until just tender.

2 Tbsp. margarine
1 clove minced garlic
¾ cup minced onion
¼ cup chopped celery

SAUTE for 5 minutes.

¼ cup chopped parsley
¼ tsp. rosemary
¼ basil
¾ tsp. salt

ADD to sauteed vegetables and simmer, covered, for 10 minutes. Toss well with beans.

SERVES 6

GREEN BEANS A LA SESAME

76 Cal. per serving

1 lb. fresh or frozen green beans

COOK until crispy tender.

2 Tbsp. sesame seeds
¼ cup slivered almonds
2 Tbsp. oil

LIGHTLY brown seeds and almonds in oil.

¼ tsp. salt
1 tsp. lemon juice

ADD to oil and pour over green beans. Toss to mix well. This sauce is good on broccoli, cauliflower, etc.

SERVES 6

YELLOW SQUASH POTATO PATTIES

70 Cal. per serving

1½ cups shredded yellow squash (unpeeled)
1 cup shredded new potatoes (unpeeled)
1 small onion, minced
2 eggs
½ cup dried bread crumbs
1 tsp. salt
¼ cup toasted wheat germ
¼ tsp. basil
¼ tsp. Italian seasoning

COMBINE all ingredients and mix thoroughly. Form into patties on greased cookie sheet. Bake at 350° till lightly browned. Serve with applesauce, hot tomato sauce or yogurt.

SERVES 8

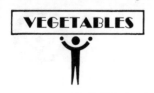

VEGETABLES

SKILLET VERMICELLI AND PEAS

176 Cal. per serving

3 Tbsp. salad oil ¼ cup margarine	HEAT in large skillet.
1-8-oz. pkg. fine vermicelli noodles ½ cup onion, chopped 1 tsp. salt 2 garlic cloves, halved	ADD and cook over medium heat. You may remove garlic halves when they are brown. Stir noodles until they are golden brown.
2½ cups seasoned broth 1 cup evaporated milk 1-10 oz. pkg. frozen peas	ADD broth, cream and peas. Cover and cook just until noodles are tender.

SERVES 4

ZUCCHINI PATTIES

140 Cal. per serving

2 large zucchini 1 onion	GRATE unpeeled zucchini and onion.
1 cup seasoned bread crumbs ½ cup wheat germ 1 egg 1 tsp. seasoned salt ground bread crumbs	MIX all ingredients. Form into patties and roll on both sides in ground crumbs. Fry until browned. Serve with brown gravy.

SERVES 6

LIMA CASSEROLE

162 Cal. per serving (with cheese)
133 Cal. per serving (without cheese)

1 lb. dry lima beans	SIMMER beans until tender; salt lightly.
2 Tbsp. oil ½ cup bell peppers, chopped ¼ cup grated onion	SAUTE green pepper and onion in oil.
1 - 4 oz. can mushrooms 1 pkg. Lipton tomato soup 1 tsp. salt ½ cup grated cheese (optional)	MEASURE liquid from mushrooms and that remaining from beans to make 1¾ cups. If there is not enough liquid, add water. Combine with remaining ingredients and bake at 350° for 30 minutes.

SERVES 8

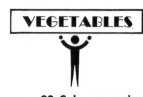
SQUASH CREOLE

92 Cal. per serving

½ cup onion, chopped
1 clove garlic, minced, optional
½ cup green pepper, chopped
2 Tbsp. oil

SAUTE onion, garlic and pepper in oil until tender.

2 Tbsp. flour
2 cups canned or cooked tomatoes

BLEND in flour. Gradually add tomatoes, mixing well. Cook over low heat.

1 tsp. sugar
½ tsp. dried basil
1 bay leaf
½ tsp. salt

ADD sugar and seasoning. Stir until thickened.

3 cups diced acorn or butternut squash

PLACE squash in greased 1½ quart casserole. Cover with sauce and bake 60 minutes at 350°. May be served over rice.

SERVES 8

DILLED YELLOW SUMMER SQUASH WITH YOGURT 85 Cal. per serving

½ cup onion, chopped
2 Tbsp. oil

SAUTE onion in oil until golden.

2 lbs. summer squash

WASH and cut unpeeled squash into quarters lengthwise, then into 2 inch lengths.

1 tsp. salt
½ tsp. paprika
1 tsp. dill seed
1 Tbsp. lemon juice
1 Tbsp. water

ADD squash, seasonings and lemon juice. Cover and simmer over low heat for 10 min., stirring occasionally until squash is tender.

2/3 cup yogurt
1 Tbsp. dried parsley

DRAIN squash if necessary. Remove from heat and stir in yogurt and parsley. DO NOT REHEAT OR YOGURT WILL CURDLE.

SERVES 6

BROILED ONION RINGS

2 large onions

CUT in ⅜ inch slices. Cook in boiling water for five minutes. Separate into rings. Pat dry.

salad oil
1½ cup finely crushed corn flakes

DIP rings in oil, then in crumbs. Place under broiler about 10 minutes.

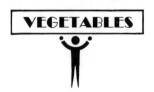

VEGETABLES

HONEY BAKED ACORN SQUASH

183 Cal. per serving

4 small acorn squash	CUT squash in half. Remove membranes and seeds.
2 cups orange juice or water	ARRANGE squash in greased 8x12 pyrex dish into which orange juice or water has been poured.
4 Tbsp. honey **4 Tbsp. oil** **¼ tsp. cinnamon** **1/3 tsp. salt**	BLEND honey, oil and seasonings together. Spoon mixture into cavities of squash or onto cut squares. Bake covered with foil at 350° for 30 minutes. Baste with orange juice, then uncover and bake another 30 min.
buttered peas	FILL with buttered peas.

ZUCCHINI AND BROWN RICE

151 Cal. per serving

1 cup brown rice **3 cups water** **1 tsp. salt**	COVER and cook rice over low heat (about 25 minutes)
3 small zucchini squash, sliced	ADD squash to rice and continue cooking for 15 minutes (until water absorbs.)
1-2 Tbsp. margarine	MIX lightly with rice and squash and serve.

SERVES 6

RATATOUILLE

64 Cal. per serving

1 medium onion, peeled & chopped **1 clove garlic, minced (optional)** **2 Tbsp. olive oil**	SAUTE onions and garlic in olive oil for 5 minutes.
2 zucchini squash, thinly sliced **1 small eggplant, peeled & cubed** **1 green pepper, cut into inch pieces**	ADD squash, eggplant and green pepper to skillet and more oil as needed. SAUTE mixture for 10 minutes, stirring gently.
2 cups stewed tomatoes, quartered **1 tsp. dried basil** **1 Tbsp. flaked dried parsley** **1 tsp. salt**	STIR in tomatoes and seasonings. Reduce heat to low, cover skillet tightly and simmer 15 minutes. Serve immediately. Good over rice.

SERVES 8

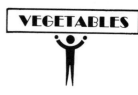

GOLDEN VEGETABLE BAKE

156 Cal. per serving

2 Tbsp. each butter and flour **1 cup scalded milk** **1 tsp. salt** **¾ tsp. paprika**	COMBINE to make a white sauce.
2 beaten eggs	STIR a little sauce into egg mixture, then add remainder.
1¾ cup cream style corn **1/3 cup chopped green** ** pepper** **2 Tbsp. chopped onion** **1½ cup grated carrots**	ADD vegetables. Pour into greated 1½" quart casserole. Bake at 350° for 50 min.
YIELD: 6 servings	VARIATION: By doubling the amounts for white sauce and leaving out the eggs, you have a product the consistency of thick soup that is a very tasty dish.

CONFETTI RICE MOLD

259 Cal. per serving

1 onion, quartered **2 cups raw carrot pieces** **1 sliced green pepper** **1 can (5 oz.) pimentos** **1 cup vegetable broth** **½ tsp. salt**	PLACE all ingredients in blender. Cover and turn motor on and off several times until vegetables are coarsely chopped. Pour into a saucepan.
½ cup brown rice, uncooked **¼ cup oil** **SERVES 4**	ADD to vegetables and cook until liquid is absorbed and rice is tender. If necessary, add a little more water. Pack into oiled 1½ quart mold for a few minutes. Unmold and serve.

CARROTS a l'ORANGE

43 Cal. per serving

4 medium carrots	WASH; cut in ¼ inch slices and place in skillet.
1 cup orange juice + cornstarch **1 Tbsp. honey** **dash salt** **SERVES 6**	ADD and simmer covered until tender.

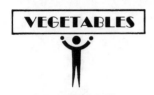

VEGETABLES

BAKED CARROTS

65 Cal. per serving

1 pound carrots

WASH, scrape and slice.

½ cup thinly sliced onion
2 Tbsp. dried parsley flakes
½ tsp. salt
1 tsp. sugar
2 Tbsp. margarine

PLACE alternate layers of carrots, onions, and seasonings in a buttered casserole. Dot with the margarine.

¼ cup boiling water

POUR over all. Cover and bake at 375° until tender.

Serves 6

BAKED CARROT RING WITH PEAS

171 Cal. per serving

1 cup thick white sauce,
   cooled
3 cups cooked mashed carrots
3 eggs
2 cups young peas

SERVES 6 generously

BEAT egg yolks till thick. Add to white sauce. Stir in mashed carrots. Fold in beaten egg whites. Bake in well buttered ring mold, set in pan of hot water. Bake at 350° for 1 hour. Remove to serving dish. Cook tender peas, season with salt and butter. Pour into center of carrot ring. Garnish with parsley. Serve hot.

CORN RING

355 Cal. per serving (with sauce)

1 ¼ cup coarse cracker crumbs
1 medium onion, chopped
¼ cup oil

COOK cracker crumbs and onion in oil until lightly browned and onion is tender.

2 eggs
1 tsp. salt
1 - 16 oz. can cream style corn
2/3 cup milk

ADD other ingredients; mix well. Pour into greased and floured ring mold. Bake at 350° for 30 minutes or until firm. Unmold on serving plate and fill center with creole sauce. (See below)

SERVES 6

CREOLE SAUCE

1 - 4 oz. can mushrooms
1 small green pepper, chopped
2 Tbsp. oil

LIGHTLY brown the drained mushrooms and chopped pepper in oil.

1 tsp. sugar
1 tsp. salt
2 tsp. cornstarch

STIR in seasonings.

1 - 16 oz. can tomatoes

ADD tomatoes; cook until thickened, stirring constantly.

SERVES 6

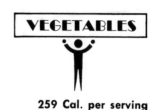

CURRIED POTATOES

259 Cal. per serving

4 medium sized potatoes
4 eggs, boiled

BOIL potatoes in salted water in skins, peel and slice. Alternate layers of potato and egg slices in greased casserole.

1-10 oz. can mushroom soup
1 cup soy "mayonnaise"
(or sour cream)
½ cup milk
1 tsp. mild curry powder
½ tsp. salt

COVER each layer of potatoes and eggs with sauce. Sprinkle top with herb seasoned crushed bread crumbs.
Bake at 350° for 30 minutes.

SERVES 6

STUFFED TOMATOES

103 Cal. per serving

6 medium tomatoes

CUT top third off in zig zag fashion. Scoop out and reserve pulp, but leave shells intact. Reserve tops.

¾ cup toasted wheat germ
1/3 cup melted margarine
½ tsp. grated lemon peel
1 Tbsp. lemon juice
1 tsp. oregano
½ tsp. onion salt

MIX together all ingredients with pulp for filling. Fill tomato shells. Place filled tomatoes in baking pan. Place reserved tops on top. Bake uncovered at 400° for 15 minutes or until hot.

SERVES 6

STUFFED MUSHROOMS

28 Cal. per mushroom

18 medium mushrooms

WASH and gently break off stems. Place in greased pan. Chop the mushroom stems.

2 Tbsp. oil

SAUTE stems in oil.

½ cup toasted wheat germ
2 Tbsp. chopped onion
2 Tbsp. minced parsley
1 Tbsp. sesame seeds
¼ tsp. crushed rosemary
¼ tsp. salt
2 Tbsp. grated cheese,
optional

COMBINE with stems. Stuff firmly into mushroom caps. Bake at 400° about 10 minutes. These are nice for hors d'oeuvres when using small mushrooms.

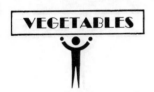

VEGETABLES

LEFTOVER POTATO PATTIES

74 Cal. per patty

1 chopped onion
2 Tbsp. oil

SAUTE onion until golden.

2 cups mashed potato, or
    any amount cold leftover

8 patties

COMBINE with sauted onion and shape into small flat patties. Roll in flour and brown both sides in oil, or bake on a greased cookie sheet in a moderate oven until brown.

HAWAIIAN YAMS

202 Cal. per serving

2 lbs. cooked yams, canned
    or fresh

SLICE yams and place in a buttered 2 quart casserole.

1 large banana

SLICE and arrange on top of yams.

½ cup orange juice

POUR juice over top.

½ tsp. salt

SPRINKLE on top.

¼ cup chopped pecans
¼ cup flaked coconut

SPRINKLE evenly over top. Bake at 350° covered for 30 minutes

SERVES 6

APPLE-YAM CASSEROLE

222 Cal. per serving

6 cold cooked yams
4 large crisp tart apples

PEEL yams and apples.

Slice and layer in buttered casserole with butter pieces and brown sugar sprinkled between each
  layer.
Bake at 350° for 1 hour. Serve hot.

SERVES 6

PINEAPPLE-BEET TREAT

116 Cal. per serving

6 medium sized beets, cooked
    and peeled

SLICE beets.

2 cups crushed pineapple
juice of one lemon
1 rounded tsp. corn starch

ADD pineapple with juice, lemon juice, mixed with corn starch. Stir over low heat until slightly thickened.

1 tsp. margarine

SERVES 6

ADD the margarine and more sweetening in the way of sugar, if needed. Simmer until hot.

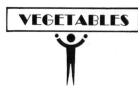

SIMPLE CABBAGE CASSEROLE

112 Cal. per serving

1 whole cabbage, cut up	PARBOIL cabbage until tender.
1 cup celery, chopped ½ cup onion, chopped ½ cup green pepper, chopped ½ can meatless burger*	SAUTE celery, onion, green pepper and burger in small amount of oil.
1 4 oz. can tomato sauce minced garlic parsley oregano, salt, Italian seasoning	ADD seasoning and tomato sauce.
½ cup shredded mild cheese SERVES 8	ALTERNATE cabbage and sauce mixture in baking dish with ½ cup mild chesse, shredded on top. Bake at 350° for 30 minutes.

CAULIFLOWER AND CHEESE CASSEROLE

282 Cal. per serving

3 cups diced cauliflower	COOK until almost done.
2 cups white sauce 1 minced green pepper 1 cup thick tomato puree	MIX while still hot with the cauliflower. Season with salt to taste. Pour into a casserole.
½ cup fine bread crumbs 1 cup grated cream cheese 2 Tbsp. melted margarine	MIX all together and spread on top of casserole mixture. Bake covered at 350° until heated through. Then remove cover and allow top to brown nicely.

SERVES 8

SPINACH SUPREME

77 Cal. per serving

2 10 oz. pkgs. frozen chopped spinach	COOK and drain spinach.
2 Tbsp. well mixed onion soup mix (dry)	WHILE hot, add dry onion soup mix. Cool.
1 cup sour cream, soy or dairy seasoned bread crumbs	ADD sour cream. Top with enough bread crumbs to cover. Bake, uncovered, at 300° for 20 minutes. Try this with other greens.

SERVES 8

*See pg. 61

Soups

MOCK CHICKEN SOUP
195 Cal. per serving

2 medium potatoes

PEEL, dice and parboil potatoes for 8 min.

¼ cup finely cut parsley
(dried)
1 stalk celery, diced
1½ cups water
½ tsp. salt
1 diced onion
2 bay leaves

ADD and simmer till tender. Mash with potato masher.

2 scrambled eggs, mashed
½ cup milk
1 Tbsp. butter
2 tsp. chicken style seasoning

ADD remaining ingredients and warm. Add enough milk for desired consistency.

SERVES 4

CHICKEN STYLE NOODLE SOUP
155 Cal. per serving

1 cup chopped onion
2 Tbsp. oil

SAUTE until golden, in large soup kettle.

8 cups water
2 diced potatoes
1-13 oz. can Soyameat, diced,
with juice
2 Tbsp. chicken style
seasoning
¼ cup chopped parsley

ADD and cook until potatoes are almost done.

1 cup thin noodles, uncooked

ADD and cook until noodles are done. Adjust salt to taste.

SERVES 10

CORN CHOWDER
110 Cal. per serving

1 cup diced raw potatoes
½ cup diced onion
½ cup diced celery
¼ cup diced green pepper
¾ cup boiling water
1 pkg. G. Washington Broth

COMBINE. Heat to boiling. Reduce heat. Simmer. Do not overcook.

1-16 oz. can cream style corn
1½ cup milk
1½ tsp. salt

ADD to previous ingredients and heat to boiling point. Serve.

SERVES 6

POTTAGE VICTORIA

169 Cal. per serving

1 large potato 2 cups corn, creamed style 1 cup asparagus, cut (frozen or canned) 2 cups water	COOK potato, corn and asparagus in water. Blend smooth in blender or grind.
2 cups cream or half & half 2 cups milk 1½ tsp. salt 1½ tsp. Accent	ADD milk, cream and seasonings.

SERVES 8

ONION POTATO SOUP

136 Cal. per serving

1 medium onion, chopped 2 potatoes, diced 2 cups water	COMBINE and cook until potato is very soft.
2 tsp. salt 2 Tbsp. margarine 1 quart milk	ADD and heat through, but do not boil.
1 tsp. parsley flakes	SPRINKLE on top when serving.

SERVES 8

DUTCH POTATO SOUP

207 Cal. per serving

1 medium sized onion, chopped 3 Tbsp. oil	SAUTE onion in oil in soup ketle.

3 medium sized potatoes,
  sliced
3 cups water (enough to
  cover)
	ADD potatoes and water. Simmer until tender.

1 cup evaporated milk 1 cup small curd cottage cheese 1 Tbsp. parsley flakes	ADD evaporated milk, bring just to a boil and gently stir in cottage cheese and parsley flakes.

SERVES 6

SOUPS

FAMOUS SPLIT PEA SOUP
100 Cal. per serving

1 lb. green split dried peas
2 quarts water
1 stalk celery, chopped
1 medium carrot, chopped
1 small onion, chopped
¾ tsp. thyme
1 bay leaf
salt to taste

SERVES 10

PLACE all ingredients in kettle and boil hard for 20 minutes. Turn down heat. Simmer until peas are soft, approximately 1 hour. Pass through colander and serve.

LENTIL SOUP
172 Cal. per serving

2 cups lentils, dry
½ cup minced onion
½ cup finely diced celery and leaves
¼ cup finely cut parsley
½ tsp. salt
1½ quarts cold water
2 cups tomatoes

PLACE in kettle. Bring slowly to boiling point and simmer for 1 hour or till tender. Add more water if necessary to prevent sticking. Mash lentils with potato masher or put through sieve.

¼ tsp. thyme
1 Tbsp. oil
1 Tbsp. butter
1 Tbsp. Vegex or soy sauce
additonal water to give desired consistency

SERVES 10

ADD remaining ingredients. Reheat and serve.

VEGETABLE SOUP
102 Cal. per serving

½ cup white navy beans
½ cup pearl barley

Boil beans and barley in 6 cups of water until tender.

2 celery stalks with leaves, chopped
1 carrot, chopped
1 onion, chopped
2 medium sized beets, chopped
2 medium sized potatoes, chopped
parsley
salt
1 pkg. G. Washington Broth (optional)

ADD remaining ingredients.

½ cup tomato juice

WHEN vegetables are nearly done, stir in tomato juice.

SERVES 10

HEARTY BEAN SOUP

269 Cal. per serving

1 lb. pkg. small navy beans	SOAK beans in hot water until softened, then cook until tender. Partially mash beans.
1 onion, minced 1 cup carrots, cubed 1 cup celery, chopped ¼ cup cumin seed ½ tsp. Accent salt to taste	ADD remaining ingredients and simmer till done.

SERVES 6

BEAN SOUP SPECIAL

223 Cal. per serving

1 pound beans, cooked	COOKED beans should not be too soft and should have at least 1 ½ quarts of water for liquid.
2 Tbsp. olive oil 1 onion, chopped 1 garlic clove, chopped 3 sprigs parsley, chopped 3 carrots, chopped 3 celery stalks, chopped 1 cup diced potatoes 1 cup shredded cabbage	SAUTE together onions, garlic, parsley, carrots, celery, potatoes and cabbage, stirring often. Add to beans.
1 cup cooked macaroni 1 Tbsp. salt 1 cup cooked tomatoes	ADD macaroni, salt and tomato. Simmer 15 minutes longer.

SERVES 8-10

YUMMY ASPARAGUS SOUP

276 Cal. per serving

1 ½ cups milk 1-10 oz. can asparagus soup	BLEND asparagus soup and milk in double boiler.
½ tsp. salt 2 Tbsp. margarine	ADD salt, butter and heat.
1 bell pepper 3 medium tomatoes	ADD bell pepper, sliced into thin round slices (seeds removed) and tomatoes cut into wedges, (about 8 wedges to a tomato). Simmer gently until vegetables are just crisply tender and serve at once.

SERVES 3

SQUASH SOUP

181 Cal. per serving

2 cups cooked winter squash, mashed
1 medium sized onion, chopped
½ tsp. sage
½ tsp. celery seed
1 tsp. parsley flakes
2 tsp. salt
3 cups water

COMBINE all ingredients in a large kettle. Cover tightly and simmer over medium heat for 30 minutes. Cool and puree in blender.

1 Tbsp. soy flour
1 Tbsp. oil
½ cup water
½ tsp. Accent
2 cups evaporated milk
1 Tbsp. parsley flakes

ADD oil to soy flour. Gradually add water, making smooth mixture. Dilute with remaining water and milk and add to puree mixture. Add Accent and parsley flakes. Heat thoroughly.

SERVES 6

CHINESE SOUP DELECTABLE

127 Cal. per serving

2 Tbsp. minced onion
2 Tbsp. margarine or oil

SAUTE onion in oil.

1 tsp. salt (or more)
2/3 cup rice, dry
3 cups cold water
2 cups potato water

ADD and cook until rice is nearly tender.

1 minced, hard-boiled egg

ADD hard-boiled egg. Serve hot.

SERVES 6

Vegetarian chicken seasoning can be added sparingly. Taste for saltiness.

QUICK BORSCHT

109 Cal. per serving

¾ cup yogurt
1 cup sour cream
1 Tbsp. lemon juice
¼ tsp. salt
¼ tsp. onion powder
1½ cups diced cooked beets

PLACE all ingredients in blender. Cover, and blend at high speed until smooth. Serve cold with an extra dollop of yogurt.

SERVES 6

RED BORSCHT

93 Cal. per serving

1 onion, chopped
2 carrots, diced
2 stalks celery, diced
½ cabbage, grated
3 potatoes, cubed
3 beets, grated
4 Tbsp. oil

SAUTE vegetables in oil in large kettle.

2 cups stewed tomatoes
3 tsp. lemon juice

ADD tomatoes and lemon juice and simmer 10 minutes.

2 quarts water
2 Tbsp. beef style seasoning
1 tsp. dill seed
salt to taste

ADD seasonings and water. Simmer until vegetables are cooked. Put a spoonful of sour cream on top of each serving of soup.

SERVES 12

HEARTY CREAMED VEGETABLE SOUP

240 Cal. per serving

4 medium sized potatoes, diced
1 onion, diced finely
1-10 oz. pkg. diced carrots (frozen)
6 cups water
2 tsp. salt

COOK until nearly done.

ADD.

1 10 oz. pkg. peas (frozen or canned)

BLEND ingredients in separate pan to make cream sauce.

¼ cup oil
½ cup flour
1 tsp. salt
½ tsp. Accent

2 cups evaporated milk

ADD, stirring constantly till thickened. Gradually add water from boiled vegetables to thin as necessary. Cook 10 minutes. Add white sauce to vegetables in remaining water and stir thoroughly. Salt to taste.

SERVES 8

SOUPS

MINESTRONE ALLA MILANESE 192 Cal. per serving

¼ cup olive oil
1 minced garlic clove
1 minced onion
1 Tbsp. chopped parsley
dash of basil

COOK in a large kettle until soft.

3 cups canned or fresh
   tomatoes
2 stalks chopped celery
2 diced carrots
2 diced potatoes
2 cups diced zucchini
1 cup shredded cabbage
2 cups cut string beans
6 cups hot water
salt to taste

ADD and simmer covered for ½ hour.

½ cup brown rice, dry

ADD and cook until done. For Southern Italian minestrone add small macaroni instead of rice.

SERVES 8

TOMATO SOUP 250 Cal. per serving

4 Tbsp. flour
4 Tbsp. oil

BLEND together as for white sauce.

1 tsp. salt
2 cups pureed tomatoes

ADD and bring to boil. Boil one minute to cook tomatoes.

2 cups hot milk

STIR above mixture into milk to avoid curdling.

SERVES 4

WORTH TRYING CABBAGE SOUP 267 Cal. per serving

2 cups cabbage, grated
½ cup blanched almonds,
   chopped
½ cup water
3 Tbsp. margarine
1 tsp. caraway seed
½ tsp. paprika
salt to taste

COOK cabbage with almonds, margarine and seasonings for 10 minutes.

1 egg, beaten
4 cups milk

ADD egg to milk and combine with cabbage mixture. Heat through, but DO NOT BOIL.

¼ cup grated cheese

TOP with grated cheese.

SERVES 6

The Latest on Fiber

What does wheat lose in the refining process?

- FIBER
- Vitamins and minerals (50-90%)
- Protein
- Desirable fat

Why is fiber important in the diet?[1]

- Shortens the passage time of bowel contents
- Absorbs water and prevents loss of fluid from colon, thereby
- PREVENTS CONSTIPATION

What diseases today result directly or indirectly from a fiber deficient, refined-food diet?

- Diverticulosis
- Appendicitis
- Colon polyps and cancer
- Hiatus hernia
- Hemorrhoids
- Coronary heart disease
- Gall stones
- Obesity
- Varicose veins

What foods have the BEST fiber content?

- Bran (1 cup/day gives adequate fiber in the diet)
- Whole wheat (3 slices of w.w. bread contains adequate fiber)
- Potatoes: Irish or yams
- Whole grain cereals
- Legumes (beans of every variety and peas)
- Dried fruits (fresh fruits contain less fiber because of high water content)
- Bananas

Try multi-grain Bran Bread recipe, page 87.

NOTE: 1 cup of unprocessed bran may be substituted for 1 cup of white or whole wheat flour in our bread recipes.

BREADS BREAKFASTS

Hearty Breakfasts - Why?

- Food is best digested early in the day
- Body needs energy for the entire day's work
- Calories at breakfast are more apt to be "exercised off" during the day
- Breakfast ideally should contain 1/3 to 1/2 of daily food requirement
- Avoid constipation by eating whole grain cereal daily. Bran is especially recommended.
- Try BRANOLA recipe, page 109.

Why do Americans often skip breakfast?

- Do not understand the importance of this meal
- Dieting
- Not hungry (due to poor habit pattern or undigested late heavy evening meal)
- Too rushed; would rather sleep late

Who skips breakfast?

- Children
  only one out of 20 children has a good breakfast
- Teen Agers
  48% of girls have no breakfast
  24% of boys leave off this meal
- Adults
  46% eat no breakfast [2]

When and How Often should one eat?

- There should be 5-6 hours between meals for most adults
- If there is a third meal, it should be eaten several hours before going to sleep, so that sleep will not be disturbed
- Excessive fats, eaten late in the day, followed by inactivity, may be deposited in the vessels, giving rise in time to hardening of the arteries.
- According to life insurance statistics, the majority of Americans are overweight, therefore —
- For adults, two meals a day, avoiding the last meal, is preferred
- Weight is more easily lost by dieters who skip supper instead of breakfast (because of usual inactivity following supper)

References:
1. Burkitt, Dr. D. P., Lecture Singapore General Hospital, Nov 4, 1975
2. Breakfast Source Book, Cereal Institute, Inc., Chicago, Ill. 1966

Breads

BASIC BREAD RECIPE

4 cups lukewarm water 3 pkgs. yeast	SPRINKLE yeast on water and stir.
1/3 cup honey 1/3 cup oil 1 Tbsp. salt 1¾ cups skimmed milk powder	ADD and stir well.
5 cups whole wheat flour	ADD and mix well.
4 to 5 cups unbleached enriched white flour	ADD 3 cups of the white flour and mix well. Turn out on a floured bread board and knead for 10 minutes, adding remaining flour a little at a time until dough is smooth and not sticky. Place in an oiled bowl. Turn once to grease top. Cover and let rise until double in bulk. Punch down. Form into 3 loaves. Let rise until double. Bake at 350° for 45 minutes. Cover loaves
3 loaves	with foil if browning too rapidly.

QUICK 100% WHOLE WHEAT BREAD

1 cup warm water 1 Tbsp. honey 2 pkgs. yeast	COMBINE in small bowl and let stand about 10 minutes.
3 cups hot water 1/3 cup honey 4 Tbsp. oil 1 Tbsp. salt 4 cups whole wheat flour	MIX in large bowl in order given. Cool to luke-warm and add yeast mixture. Beat thoroughly in electric mixer or vigorously by hand. Let this rise in a warm place 15 minutes.
Approx. 5 cups whole wheat flour warmed in a 250° oven	ADD enough warm flour to make soft dough which can be handled. Knead 5 minutes. Throw the mass of dough with force onto the bread board several times. Put in loaves into well greased pans and allow to sit for 12 minutes. Bake at 250° for 15 minutes. Increase heat to
3 loaves	350° and finish baking about 45 minutes.

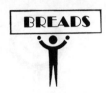

FORTIFIED WHITE BREAD

3 cups milk	SCALD and cool till lukewarm.
2 pkgs. yeast 2 Tbsp. honey	SPRINKLE yeast in milk, add honey, and let stand 5 minutes.
6 cups unbleached enriched flour ½ cup soy flour ¾ cup powdered milk 4 tsp. salt	SIFT together. Add half of the flour mixture to the milk and beat with egg beater or electric mixer till smooth.
2 Tbsp. oil ¼ cup wheat germ 2-3 loaves	ADD; stir in rest of flour mixture to make a stiff dough. Knead 5 minutes till smooth and elastic. Put in oiled bowl, turn to oil top and cover with a damp cloth. Let rise until double. Punch down and let rise again. Punch down. Form into Loaves. Let rise. Bake at 350° about 50 minutes.

BOB'S BREAD

4 cups warm water 3 pkgs. (3 Tbsp.) dry yeast	DISSOLVE yeast in water.
½ cup brown sugar 2 Tbsp. salt ½ cup oil (or more)	ADD to above and mix.
6 cups whole wheat flour 6 cups white flour	WHEN adding flour to above ingredients, alternate whole wheat then white till you reach desired consistency. Use as little flour as possible for moister bread.
	KNEAD 10-15 minutes. Round in large greased bowl. Oil top and place damp cloth over it to keep from forming dry crust. Set in warm place, (80-90°F) about 1½ hours or until dough doubles.
3-4 loaves	DIVIDE into 3 or 4 loaves. Place in greased pans. Let it stand for ½ hour covered with damp cloth. Bake at 350° for 45 minutes.

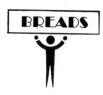
MULTI-GRAIN BRAN BREAD

½ cup warm water
3 pkgs. yeast

SPRINKLE yeast over water to dissolve.

4 cups warm water
2 Tbsp. sugar
1 cup bran, unprocessed
1 cup wheat germ
1 cup oatmeal
1 cup rye flour
2 cups unbleached enriched
   white flour

ADD to yeast and beat well to make a sponge.
Let rise until bubbly, about 30 minutes.

2 Tbsp. salt
6 Tbsp. oil
¾ cup honey
4 cups whole wheat flour
   approx. 2 cups white flour

ADD to make a stiff dough and knead till
smooth. Cover; let rise till double in bulk. Punch
down. Form into loaves or rolls. Let rise again
until double. Bake at 350° 45 minutes to one
hour.

4 loaves

MARVELOUS OATMEAL BREAD

2 cups quick oats
½ cup oil
½ cup sugar
¼ cup sorghum or molasses
1 Tbsp. salt

MIX in very large bowl.

2 cups boiling water

POUR over mixture.

4 Tbsp. dry yeast
½ cup warm water

DISSOLVE yeast in water.

2 cups cold water

ADD to first mixture; then add yeast.

½ cup wheat germ
½ cup soy flour
2 cups whole wheat flour
6 cups unbleached enriched
   flour

ADD and knead. Place in oiled bowl. Turn to
oil top. Let rise till double. Punch down. Form
into loaves. Put in pans; let rise till double.
Bake at 350° for 40 minutes.

3 loaves

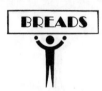

BREADS

NO FAIL OATMEAL BREAD

2 cups quick oats
¾ cup oil
¼ cup brown sugar
¼ cup molasses
1 Tbsp. salt

MIX together in a very large bowl.

2 cups boiling water

ADD to above and stir well.

2 cups cold water

ADD and stir well again.

3 pkgs. yeast, dissolved in
  ½ cup warm water

ADD and mix well.

½ cup wheat germ
2 cups whole wheat flour
approx. 6 cups unbleached
  enriched white flour

ADD wheat germ and flour until it becomes difficult to mix, then turn out on a floured board. Knead in remaining flour until smooth. Place dough in greased bowl; let rise in a warm place until double in bulk. Turn out on board and knead down. Form into loaves and place in greased pans about half full. Allow dough to rise only to the top of the pans. Bake at 375° about 45 minutes. Cool on racks and brush tops with margarine.

3 loaves

OATMEAL FRUIT BREAD

1 pkg. yeast
½ cup warm water

ADD yeast to water and let soften.

1 cup hot water
1 Tbsp. oil
½ tsp. salt
½ cup oatmeal

MIX hot water, oil, salt, oatmeal, and set aside to cool to lukewarm. Combine with yeast mixture.

2 Tbsp. molasses
2 Tbsp. brown sugar
½ cup unbleached enriched
  flour

ADD to make a sponge. Stir until smooth. Cover with a towel and let stand in a warm place away from drafts about 10 minutes.

¼ cup raisins
½ cup dried, chopped
  apricots

WASH and drain fruit and add to sponge.

2 cups whole wheat flour
approx. 1 cup unbleached
  flour

ADD flour till stiff enough to knead. Knead 10 minutes. Shape into ball, grease top and put in greased bowl. Cover and let rise till double. Punch down. Shape into loaf and place in greased pan, turning to grease top. Let rise till double. Bake at 400° for 10 minutes and 45 minutes at 325°.

1 loaf

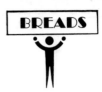

NO KNEAD OATMEAL BREAD

2 cups boiling water
1 cup rolled oats
1/3 cup oil
½ cup light molasses
1 Tbsp. salt

COMBINE in a large bowl and let cool until lukewarm.

2 pkgs. yeast
2 eggs, optional

ADD when above mixture is lukewarm. Beat well.

½ cup rye flour
½ cup soy flour
½ cup wheat germ
2 cups whole wheat flour
about 2 cups unbleached enriched flour

ADD flour gradually, beating well after each addition. You may substitute if you don't have rye or soy flour. Mix until well blended to make a moderately stiff dough. Grease top and cover bowl. Store in refrigerator at least 2 hours or overnight. Turn out on floured surface. Punch down and shape into 2 loaves. Place in greased bread pans. Grease tops and let rise in a warm place until double (about 2 hours). Bake at 350° about 45 minutes. If crust browns too fast cover with foil for last half of baking. The dough may also be made into rolls. Rolls bake in 25 minutes.

2 loaves

FLOURLESS SPROUTED WHEAT BREAD

1 lb. dry wheat kernels

SOAK in warm water for about 4 hours. Drain and allow to sprout for about 20 more hours. This works well in a large jar. Lay it on its side so that a small amount of water remains. You will see tiny white sprouts starting. Rinse the wheat with cool water. Grind wheat very fine, twice.

1 Tbsp. soft margarine
2 Tbsp. brown sugar

ADD to ground wheat.

1 pkg. yeast
2 Tbsp. warm water

DISSOLVE yeast in water and add. Knead for a few minutes on a floured board. Shape into a loaf and place in a well greased pan. Allow to rise until double (about 1 hour). Bake at 375° for 40 to 50 minutes.

1 loaf

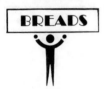

BREADS

MOTHER'S STIRRED GRAHAM BREAD

2 pkgs. yeast
5 cups warm water

COMBINE and let stand 10 minutes.

2 Tbsp. brown sugar
2 cups bran
2 Tbsp. salt
1 cup wheat germ
5 cups unbleached enriched
white flour
4 cups whole wheat flour
2 cups chopped nuts -
optional
2 cups raisins - optional

ADD to yeast mixture and stir thoroughly. Put in greased pans and let rise till nearly double in bulk.

BAKE at 350° for 45 minutes to 1 hour until done.

4 loaves

SPROUTED WHEAT BREAD

1 cup wheat kernels

COVER with water and soak overnight. Drain and keep in colander about 12 hours, rinsing occasionally and cover with a damp towel.

2 pkgs. yeast
½ cup warm water
1 tsp. sugar

COMBINE and let stand 10 minutes.

2 cups warm water

TAKE the wheat, which will have tiny white sprouts showing, and will now measure about 2 cups, and blend in blender using half the wheat and half the water at a time. Add to yeast mixture.

2 Tbsp. molasses
2 tsp. salt
2 Tbsp. oil
approx. 5 cups whole wheat
flour

ADD to above and mix well. Use enough flour to make a medium soft dough. Knead until smooth. Place in greased bowl and let rise till double. Punch down and let rise again. Shape into loaves and let rise until double. Bake at 350° about one hour.

2 loaves

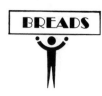

PUMPERNICKEL BREAD

2 pkgs. yeast
½ cup warm water
1 tsp. sugar

SPRINKLE yeast on water and sugar and stir to dissolve.

2 cups hot water
2 Tbsp. dark molasses
2 cups whole wheat flour
2 cups rye flour

MIX together and beat vigorously. Add yeast mixture and mix again.

2 tsp. salt
2 Tbsp. oil
2 tsp. powdered caraway seed
about 2 cups unbleached
enriched white flour

2 loaves

ADD, using enough flour to make a stiff dough. Knead until smooth. Place in an oiled bowl. Turn to oil top of dough. Cover and let rise until double. Punch down. Form into loaves. Place loaves on a greased cookie sheet. Let rise until double. Put pan of hot water on bottom rack of oven, with loaves on rack above. Bake at 350° about 45 minutes until done.

POTATO BREAD

1 medium potato
1 quart water

GRATE potato directly into 1 quart water. Boil until potato is done.

1 Tbsp. sugar

ADD sugar and allow mixture to cool.

2 pkgs. yeast
1 Tbsp. salt
1 Tbsp. shortening

ADD yeast when lukewarm. Add salt and shortening.

10 cups flour

3 loaves

BEAT in enough flour so you can handle dough to knead for 10 minutes. Let rise until double in bulk. Knead down and let rise again, (may be omitted if time is short). Mold into loaves and put into greased pans. Bake for 50 minutes at 350°.

HERB BREAD

Use your favorite bread dough recipe. When ready to form into loaves, roll out and brush with melted shortening. Sprinkle with parsley flakes, oregano, basil, onion flakes, and garlic salt, or use your favorite herbs. Roll up tightly and place in bread pans. Bake as usual.

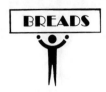

WHOLE WHEAT CARROT BREAD

1 pkg. yeast
¼ cup warm water

ADD yeast to water and let soften about 10 minutes.

1½ cups warm water
¼ cup molasses
2 cups unbleached enriched
    flour

COMBINE with yeast mixture. Beat until well mixed. Let rise until bubbly, (about 30 minutes).

3 medium carrots - about
    2 cups
1 cup warm water

BLEND carrots with water in blender or grate fine and combine with water. Add to yeast sponge.

4 Tbsp. oil
1 Tbsp. salt
7-8 cups whole wheat flour

ADD making a very stiff dough. Knead on a well floured board for 10 minutes. Place in oiled bowl, turning dough to oil on top. Cover; let rise till double in bulk. Punch down. Let rise till double again. Shape into loaves or rolls. Let rise until double. Bake at 400° for 10 minutes. Reduce to 350° for 45 minutes.

3 medium sized loaves

TOMATO BREAD

2 cups tomato puree or juice
2 Tbsp. oil
2 tsp. salt
½ cup honey or brown sugar

PLACE tomato juice, oil, salt and sugar or honey in pan and warm it.

2/3 cups warm water
2 pkgs. yeast

IN separate bowl, sprinkle yeast on warm water. Let stand 10 minutes. Then add to tomato mixture.

3 cups unbleached enriched
    white flour
3½ cups whole wheat
    flour (approx.)

ADD 3 cups white flour and mix until smooth. Add 3½ cups whole wheat flour, or little less if it would be too stiff. Knead for about 10 minutes, by the clock. Let rise in warm place until double in bulk. Cut in half. Let stand ten minutes. Shape into two loaves. Let rise until double in bulk. Bake 15 minutes at 400° and then 45 minutes to one hour at 350°.

2 loaves

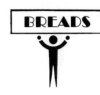

BREADS

ONION BREAD

1½ cups warm water 1 pkg. yeast	SPRINKLE yeast over water in a large bowl. Stir to dissolve.
1 Tbsp. dry minced onion 2 Tbsp. sugar 2 Tbsp. oil 2 tsp. seasoned salt ½ cup wheat germ 1½ cups unbleached enriched flour	ADD to dissolved yeast. Beat at medium speed in electric mixer for two minutes or 300 strokes by hand.
1½ cups unbleached enriched flour	ADD by hand. Let rise in warm place about 1 hour until double in bulk. Beat with spoon about 30 seconds. Spread in a greased 9x5x3 loaf pan. Pat top into shape with a floured hand. Cover with towel and let rise about 10 minutes, or until batter is about ½ inch from top of pan.
1 medium onion, sliced 2 Tbsp. melted margarine	SEPARATE onion into rings. Dip each ring in melted margarine and place on top of loaf. Bake at 375° for 35 to 40 minutes.
1 large loaf	

SWEET POTATO BREAD

1 pkg. yeast ¼ cup warm water	DISSOLVE yeast in warm water.
½ tsp. salt 3 Tbsp. oil 1½ cups mashed sweet potatoes 2 Tbsp. maple syrup 1 cup whole wheat flour	ADD to dissolved yeast. Mix well to make a smooth sponge. Cover and set in a warm place to rise about 30 minutes.
1½ to 2 cups whole wheat flour	ADD enough flour to make an elastic dough. Cover and let rise until about double. Punch down. Mold into loaves. Put in greased pans and allow to double. Bake at 350° 30 to 40 minutes.
2 small loaves	

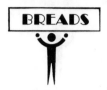

POTATO RYE BREAD

1 medium potato

PEEL thinly and boil until done. Mash finely and add the potato water to it to make 2 cups. If there is not enough water, add some from the tap.

¼ cup warm water
2 pkgs. yeast

PLACE water in a large bowl. Sprinkle yeast in and stir to dissolve.

2 Tbsp. molasses
2 Tbsp. oil
1 Tbsp. salt

ADD along with the potato and water to the dissolved yeast. Mix well.

2 cups rye flour
4 cups unbleached enriched flour
2 Tbsp. caraway seeds

ADD and stir until well mixed. Turn out on floured board and knead until soft and pliable. Place in oiled bowl. Turn to oil top. Cover and let rise in a warm place for about one hour. Punch down. Divide in half. Knead slightly, then place in greased loaf pans. Cover and let rise until almost double. Bake at 400° 45-50 minutes until done. Bread sounds hollow when tapped on the bottom when it is done.

2 loaves

BAGELS

1 cup milk

SCALD

¼ cup margarine
1½ Tbsp. sugar
½ tsp. salt

ADD to milk and let mixture cool until luke-warm.

1 pkg. yeast

ADD to lukewarm mixture.

1 egg, separated

BEAT white well and add.

3 cups flour, approximately

¼ cup wheat germ

ADD and mix well. Knead on a floured board. Cover and let rise about one hour. Roll out in small pieces, finger width and two fingers long. Shape into rings, pinching ends together well. Let stand on floured board only until they begin to rise, about 10 minutes. Drop bagels, one at a time, into a pan of hot water, just under boiling. Cook on each side approximately one minute. Place on a baking sheet.

1 tsp. cold water

BEAT water with the reserved egg yolk. Brush on bagels. Bake at 400° about 20 minutes.

1 dozen

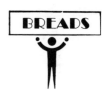

YEAST CORN BREAD

2 cups milk	SCALD and cool till lukewarm.
1 pkg. yeast **2 Tbsp. brown sugar**	SPRINKLE over milk to dissolve.
4 Tbsp. oil **2½ cups corn meal** **1½ cups sifted flour** **1 tsp. salt** **2 beaten eggs**	ADD and beat well. Fill muffin tins or shallow pan about 2/3 full. Let rise in a warm place for 1 hour. Bake at 350° about 25 minutes.

2 small loaves

ANADAMA BREAD

3 cups milk **1 cup yellow corn meal**	SCALD milk. Remove from heat and gradually add corn meal, stirring constantly. Continue to stir until mixture is smooth and thick.
½ cup molasses **2 Tbsp. margarine** **2 tsp. salt**	STIR in until well blended. Place in mixing bowl and set aside to cool to lukewarm.
2 pkgs. yeast **½ cup warm water**	DISSOLVE yeast in water and add to cornmeal when it is lukewarm.
4 cups whole wheat flour	ADD gradually and beat until very smooth.
3-4 cups unbleached enriched flour	STIR in enough white flour to make a soft dough. Turn out on a floured board. Allow to rest 5-10 min. Knead 6-8 minutes. Place in oiled bowl, turn to oil top, cover and let rise until double. Punch down. Form into loaves. Brush tops with melted margarine. Let rise until double.
3 loaves	Bake 50-60 min. at 350°. Cool on wire rack.

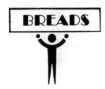

MILLET HONEY-NUT BREAD

½ cup millet
2 cups water
½ tsp. salt

COOK millet in salted water for 30 minutes.

2 pkg. yeast
½ cup water

SOFTEN yeast in water in a large bowl. When cooked millet is cooled to warm temperature, add to yeast.

¼ cup oil
1 tsp. salt
1 cup water
¼ cup honey
1 cup nuts, chopped

STIR in liquid ingredients.

5 cups whole wheat flour
   (can substitute half white
   flour)

2 loaves

STIR in flour, kneading last amount a little at a time for about 10 minutes. Let rise in greased bowl until doubled. Punch down and form into two loaves in greased bread pans. Let rise till doubled. Bake at 425° for 15 minutes, reduce heat to 350° and cover tops with foil for remaining 30 minutes of baking.

STEAMED DATE BREAD

2 pkgs. yeast
2 cups water, warm
¾ cup molasses

SOFTEN yeast in water and molasses. Let stand for a few minutes.

1 cup whole wheat flour
1 cup cornmeal
½ cup wheat germ
¼ cup soy flour

STIR into yeast mixture.

½ cup raisins
½ cup nuts, chopped
1 cup dates, chopped
1 tsp. salt

ADD fruits, nuts and salt together to batter and beat thoroughly to make light and well mixed. Pour into greased round cans and steam for 2 hours.

2 loaves

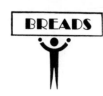

APPLE DATE ROLL

2 cups warm water
2 pkgs. yeast
½ cup honey or brown sugar

SPRINKLE yeast on water and sweetening and stir. Let rest until bubbly.

1 apple or 1 cup apples

PEEL and cube. Boil with 2 tablespoons of water for 10 minutes.

1 cup chopped dates
¾ cup water
¼ tsp. salt

SIMMER until dates dissolve and a paste is formed. Combine with apples and let cool.

¾ cup chopped nuts
    (optional)

ADD to fruit mixture.

¼ cup oil
2 tsp. salt
¼ cup soy flour
¼ cup wheat germ
5 to 7 cups white enriched
    flour

2 loaves

ADD to yeast mixture and knead until smooth. Place in oiled bowl. Turn to oil top of dough. Cover and let rise until double. Divide dough in half and roll out each half. Spread each with half of fruit mixture. Roll up tightly and place in loaf pan, or slice like cinnamon rolls. Let rise until almost double. Bake at 350° for 30 to 40 minutes.

EASY DATE NUT BREAD

3¾ cups warm water
3 pkgs. dry yeast

COMBINE and let stand 5 minutes.

6 Tbsp. oil
2 Tbsp. salt
5 cups whole wheat flour

ADD to yeast mixture. Beat at a medium speed on electric mixer for 2 minutes or 300 strokes by hand, vigorously.

1 cup chopped nuts
1¾ cups chopped dates
4 cups whole wheat or un-
    bleached white enriched
    flour

3 loaves

ADD remaining ingredients and blend with spoon until smooth. Cover, let rise till double. Stir down and spread in greased loaf pans. Batter will be sticky. Smooth out top of loaf by flouring hand and patting down. Let rise till double. Bake at 375° about 45 minutes.

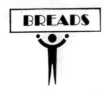

DATE-NUT BREAD

2 cups water
2 Tbsp. yeast
¼ cup brown sugar or honey

DISSOLVE yeast in water and brown sugar. Let stand until bubbly.

1/3 cup oil
1 Tbsp. salt
¼ cup soy flour
¼ cup wheat germ
2 cups whole wheat flour
3-5 cups white enriched flour

COMBINE ingredients with yeast mixture. Use just enough flour to make a medium soft dough.

2 cups chopped dates
1½ cups nuts

2 loaves

ADD dates and nuts and knead. Place in oiled bowl. Turn to oil top. Let rise till double. Punch down. Form into loaves. Put in pans; let rise till double. Bake at 350° for 40 minutes.

PRUNE-DATE WHOLE WHEAT BREAD

1 cup water
2 Tbsp. yeast
¼ cup brown sugar or honey

DISSOLVE yeast in water and brown sugar. Let stand until bubbly.

1 cup boiling water
1 cup chopped dates
1 cup chopped prunes

Allow dried fruit to soften in hot water until lukewarm.

1/3 cup oil
1 Tbsp. salt
¼ cup soy flour
¼ cup wheat germ
2 cups whole wheat flour
3-5 cups white flour
1 cup chopped nuts

COMBINE ingredients with yeast mixture. Use just enough flour to make a medium soft dough.

ADD and knead. Place in oiled bowl. Turn to oil top. Let rise till double. Punch down. Form into loaves. Put in pans; let rise till double. Bake at 350° for 40 minutes.

2 loaves

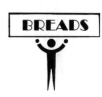

GOLDEN RAISIN-NUT SQUASH BREAD

1 cup milk	SCALD milk.
1 cup cooked winter squash, mashed ¼ cup oil ¼ cup honey 2 tsp. salt 1 tsp. cinnamon 1 tsp. ground cardamom	STIR in. Cool to lukewarm.
2 pkgs. dry yeast ½ cup warm water	SPRINKLE yeast on warm water in large bowl. Stir to dissolve. When milk mixture is lukewarm, add to yeast.
3 cups unbleached enriched flour 2 eggs 1½ cups seedless raisins ½ cup nuts, chopped	ADD 3 cups flour to mixture, then eggs, one at a time and beat until the batter is smooth. Add raisins and nuts and mix thoroughly.
3½ cups flour, (approximately) 2 loaves	MIX in enough remaining flour, a little at a time, first with a spoon, then with hands to make dough that leaves the sides of the bowl. Turn onto floured board. Knead 10 minutes until elastic. Place in greased bowl. Cover and allow to rise until doubled, about 1 hour. Punch down and turn onto board. Divide in half and shape into loaves. Place in two greased 9x5x3 pans. Brush tops with melted margarine. Cover and let rise till doubled, about 1 hour. Bake at 375° for 40 minutes.

APPLESAUCE BREAD

2 Tbsp. yeast 1 cup water	DISSOLVE.
2 cups warm applesauce ¼ cup sugar ¼ cup oil 1 tsp. salt 1 cup nuts ¼ cup soy flour ½ cup wheat germ 4½ to 5½ cups unbleached enriched white flour 2 loaves	STIR in and knead. Place in oiled bowl. Turn to oil top. Let rise till double. Punch down. Form into loaves. Put in pans; let rise till double. Bake at 375° for 20 minutes, then at 350° for 20 minutes or until done.

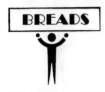

ORANGE RAISIN BREAD

1 cup raisins
2 cups reconstituted frozen orange juice

Add raisins to orange juice and heat to plump fruit. Do not boil.

¼ cup honey
1 Tbsp. grated orange rind
2 tsp. salt
2 Tbsp. oil

Put orange juice & raisins in large mixing bowl and add honey, orange rind, salt and oil. Allow to cool to warm temperature.

2 pkgs. yeast
7 cups unbleached, enriched flour

2 loaves

Dissolve yeast in warm mixture. Then gradually add flour, but keep dough soft. Knead well on board. Transfer to oiled bowl. Allow to raise double, then shape into two loaves and after second rising, bake 45 minutes at 350°F. Butter crust while still warm.

WHOLE WHEAT COTTAGE CHEESE ROLLS

1 ½ cups unbleached enriched white flour
2 pkgs. yeast

STIR flour and yeast together in large bowl.

1 ½ cups cream style cottage cheese
½ cup water
¼ cup brown sugar
2 Tbsp. margarine
2 tsp. salt

HEAT together in saucepan - cheese, water, sugar, margarine and salt till warm (not boiling), stirring constantly. Cool if necessary to lukewarm. Add to dry mixture.

2 eggs

ADD eggs and beat at low speed with mixer for ½ minute. Beat 3 minutes at high speed.

2 ½ cups whole wheat flour

1 ½ dozen rolls

BY HAND, stir in enough remaining flour to make a moderately stiff dough. Knead until smooth 8-10 minutes. Place in greased bowl, turning once. Cover; let rise till double. Punch down. Shape into rolls. Let rise till double. Bake at 375° for 12-15 minutes.

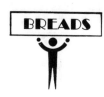

CORNMEAL ROLLS

3 cups boiling water	PLACE in top of double boiler.
1 cup cold water **1½ cups yellow cornmeal**	MIX together and stir into the boiling water. Continue cooking for 10 minutes.
1/3 cup brown sugar or honey **1/3 cup oil**	ADD to hot cornmeal. Set aside to cool.
2 pkgs. yeast **¼ cup warm water**	COMBINE and let stand until cornmeal is lukewarm. Add to cornmeal mixture.
½ cup soy flour **2 cups unbleached enriched white flour**	ADD to make a batter. Let stand until light and bubbly.
3-4 more cups of flour	ADD enough to make a soft dough. Knead thoroughly but lightly, adding as little flour as possible. Keep the dough soft. Place in oiled bowl and let rise until double. Punch down. Divide the dough into two portions. Form into rolls of desired shape. Place on greased cookie sheet and let rise until double. Bake at 375°
2 dozen rolls	for 20-25 minutes.

POTATO ROLLS

1 pkg. yeast **1 tsp. honey** **½ cup warm water** **2 Tbsp. flour**	MIX and let the batter get spongy and bubbly.
1 cup warm mashed potatoes **2 Tbsp. oil** **2 Tbsp. whole corn meal** **1½ tsp. salt** **¼ cup wheat germ** **2-3 cups unbleached enriched flour**	ADD to sponge. Knead lightly. Put in muffin tins or roll out and cut into rounds. Dough should be soft. Let rise till double in bulk. Bake 25 minutes at 350°.

1 dozen rolls

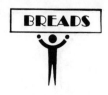

BREADS

MEDITERRANEAN POCKET BREAD

2 pkgs. yeast
2 cups warm water
1 Tbsp. brown sugar
2 cups unbleached enriched flour

COMBINE in order given and beat until smooth, about three minutes.

¼ cup oil
2 tsp. salt

ADD and mix well

3 to 4 cups whole wheat flour

ADD to make a medium stiff dough. Knead on a floured board until smooth, 5 to 10 minutes. Cover dough with bowl and let rest 30 minutes. Roll into a 16 inch log; cut into 16 pieces and shape into balls. Roll out into 5 inch circles. Place on greased baking sheets. Let rise 30-45 minutes until puffy. Bake at **500°** on bottom rack about 10 minutes. Remove and cover while cooling. Cut pocket in bread and fill with your favorite filling.

16 loaves

INDIAN CHAPATTIS

2 Tbsp. oil
1½ cups whole wheat flour
1 tsp. salt

MIX thoroughly, the flour, salt and oil.

½ to ¾ cup cold water

ADD enough water to make a soft breadlike dough. Divide into 8 balls and roll out thin. It will be about 8 inches in diameter. Bake on a hot griddle or skillet a few minutes on each side. May be spread with margarine and filled with rice, beans, or any desired filling and rolled up, or eaten as is.

8 chapattis

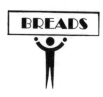

BROWN OATMEAL ROLLS

1 pkg. yeast
1/3 cup warm water
1 tsp. molasses

COMBINE yeast with warm water and sweetening and let stand 10 minutes.

1 cup quick oats
2 cups boiling water

POUR boiling water over oats and stir. Let cool.

½ cup brown sugar
2 tsp. salt
3 Tbsp. oil

ADD to oats, and then add yeast mixture.

½ cup soy flour
½ cup wheat germ
½ cup whole wheat flour
4 to 4½ cups unbleached
   enriched flour

ADD flours to make a medium soft dough. Knead lightly. Let rise. Punch down. Let rise again. Shape into rolls. Dip tops of rolls in water and into sesame seeds. Let rise till double. Bake at 375° for 20 minutes.

2 dozen rolls

WHEAT PUFFS

2 cups warm water
4 pkgs. yeast
1/3 cup honey
2 tsp. salt
3 Tbsp. melted margarine
1 cup wheat germ
4 cups whole wheat flour

COMBINE ingredients in order given. Beat well. Half fill greased muffin pans with batter. Allow to rise in a warm place until pans are full. Bake at 375° for 20-25 minutes.

2 dozen

SESAME STICKS

¼ cup sugar
¾ to 1 cup whole wheat flour
2 cups oatmeal
½ cup sesame
1 cup cashews, chopped fine
   or ground
1/3 cup oil
2/3 cup water
1 tsp. vanilla
2 tsp. salt

COMBINE all ingredients and mix thoroughly to make stiff dough. Knead into smooth ball. Divide and roll out ¼ inch thick on cookie sheet. Cut into strips 1" x 3". Bake 20-25 minutes at 350° until golden brown. If browning too fast, lower temperature and increase time. Should be crisp like crackers.

6 dozen

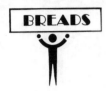

CORN MEAL TORTILLAS

½ cup yellow cornmeal ½ cup cold water	MIX together.
1 cup boiling water 1 tsp. salt	STIR cornmeal mixture into salted boiling water. Keep stirring over the heat until thick. Remove from heat and put in a bowl.
¼ cup oil	ADD and mix thoroughly.
1 cup whole wheat flour 1 cup unbleached enriched white flour 18 tortillas	STIR in gradually to make a soft dough. Use additional flour to knead. Knead till smooth. Divide into 18 equal portions. Roll each into a ball. Flatten, and roll out thin on a floured board. Bake on a hot ungreased skillet until lightly browned on both sides.

COCONUT WHEAT STICKS

1 cup unbleached enriched white flour ½ cup soy flour ½ cup whole wheat flour 1 cup coconut 1 tsp. salt 1 tsp. grated lemon peel 3 Tbsp. brown sugar	MIX thoroughly first seven ingredients.
½ cup margarine	CUT margarine into above mixture, as for pastry.
2-4 Tbsp. water 5-6 dozen	ADD water to mixture gradually, and mix thoroughly. Press into greased cookie sheet ¼ to ½ inch thick. Bake at 400° 10-12 minutes until golden brown. Cut into sticks.

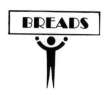

SCOTTISH OAT CRISPS

2 cups warm water
1 Tbsp. molasses
1 pkg. yeast

COMBINE in a large bowl.

3 cups oats, ground to flour
in blender
1 tsp. salt

SIFT over yeast mixture in bowl, mixing well.

2 cups flour, may be any
combination of whole
wheat and unbleached
enriched

SIFT in wheat flour until dough is not sticky and can be kneaded in bowl. Form into soft ball and cover. Let rise until double. Turn out on board. Flatten to ¾ inch and cut out rounds with a glass. Roll each round very thin. Place on greased baking sheet and let rise 30 minutes. Bake at 350° until delicate and brown and crisp. Delicious with butter, peanut butter, marmalade, or plain with salad. You may use part of recipe for regular loaf of bread.

20 rounds

BREAD STICKS

1 pkg. yeast
1¼ cups warm water
2 Tbsp. sugar

COMBINE and let stand about 10 minutes to soften.

1½ tsp. salt
1 Tbsp. margarine
½ cup wheat germ
about 3 cups unbleached
enriched flour

ADD to yeast mixture until stiff. Knead on floured board about 10 minutes until smooth. Put in oiled bowl, turn to grease top, and cover. Let rise till doubled, about 1 hour. Punch down and divide in half. Roll each half into a rectangle 12 inches long. Cut each into 12 pieces. Roll each piece to form a rope about 1/3 inch thick and 12 inches long.

sesame seed, optional
caraway seed, optional
coarse salt, optional

If desired, roll in coarse salt, sesame seed, or caraway seed. Put on greased cookie sheet, cover and let rise until double, about 1 hour. Bake 15-20 minutes at 400°.

24 sticks

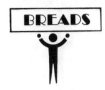

BREADS

CRISPY CRACKERS

3 cups quick oatmeal
2 cups whole wheat flour
1 cup wheat germ
1 tsp. salt
¼ cup brown sugar
½ cup sesame seeds
½ cup coconut, fine

MIX dry ingredients together.

¾ cup oil
1 cup water

BEAT oil and water and add to above mixture. Roll out on two lightly greased, large (13x17) cookie sheets. Cut in squares or diamonds. Sprinkle with salt if desired. Bake in 300° for 30 minutes or until golden brown.

6 dozen

SESAME CRACKERS

6 Tbsp. oil
½ cup water

EMULSIFY oil and water by beating with an egg beater or whizzing in blender.

2 cups whole wheat flour
½ tsp. salt

COMBINE with oil and water. Knead for 5 minutes. Let rest 10 minutes. Divide in half and roll each half on a well greased cookie sheet.

sesame seeds
additional salt

SPRINKLE with sesame seeds and salt. Roll lightly again to press in seeds. Mark in squares and prick each with a fork. Bake at 350° for ten minutes.

2 dozen

GRANOLA BREAKFAST BARS

2 cups quick oats
1 cup whole wheat flour
¼ cup soy flour
¼ cup powdered milk
¼ cup wheat germ
¼ cup rye flour
2 Tbsp. brown sugar
¼ cup honey
1 tsp. salt

MIX all together. If you don't have all the kinds of flour, you may substitute to get the same measurements.

½ cup oil

DRIZZLE over dry ingredients, and mix thoroughly about 5 minutes. Let stand ½ hour or overnight.

½ cup milk
½ cup shredded coconut

ADD. Shape into bars one quarter inch thick. Bake on greased cookie sheet at 400° 12 to 15 minutes.

3 dozen

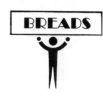
OAT CRACKERS

1/3 cup oil 1 Tbsp. honey 1 cup water	PLACE oil and honey in bowl. Gradually add water; beating to emulsify.
1 tsp. salt 3¾ cups oatmeal ¼ cup flour	ADD and mix well. Roll out on greased cookie sheet. Cut in squares. Bake at 350° for about 15 minutes. Watch carefully.

4 dozen

WHOLE WHEAT CRACKERS

6 Tbsp. oil 2/3 cup cold water	BEAT to emulsify
2 cups whole wheat flour ½ cup enriched white flour 1 cup oatmeal 1½ tsp. salt 2 Tbsp. brown sugar	MIX and add to water and oil. Roll out, cut in squares and prick with fork. Bake at 350°. Watch carefully to prevent burning.

4 dozen

OATMEAL-WHEAT CRACKERS

3 cups quick oats 2 cups whole wheat flour ½ cup enriched white flour ½ cup wheat germ 2 tsp. salt 3 Tbsp. sugar	COMBINE
¾ cup oil 1 cup water	BEAT to emulsify. Add to dry ingredients. Roll out, cut in squares, and bake at 350° for 15-20 minutes.

6 dozen

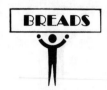

BREADS

BLUEBERRY MUFFINS

1 cup warm water 1 pkg. yeast 2 Tbsp. honey	COMBINE and let stand until foamy, about 5 minutes.
2 Tbsp. oil 2 cups whole wheat flour 1 tsp. salt	ADD and mix well.
1 cup blueberries	ADD carefully so as not to mash. Fill muffin tins half full. Let raise until up to the top. Bake at 350° until brown, about 20 minutes.

1 dozen

DATE MUFFINS

1 pkg. yeast ¼ cup warm water 1 tsp. honey	DISSOLVE yeast in warm water combined with honey and let stand about 10 minutes.
1 cup quick oats ½ tsp. salt 1 cup hot water 1¾ cup whole wheat flour ¾ cup chopped dates ¼ cup oil	ADD in order given. Mix thoroughly and beat until smooth. Put into oiled muffin tins until half full. Let rise until double. Bake at 350° about 20 minutes.

One dozen

CORN DODGERS

1 cup oats 1 cup corn meal ¼ cup soymilk powder ¼ cup sesame seed	COMBINE all dry ingredients.
¼ cup honey 2 Tbsp. oil ½ tsp. salt 1 cup hot water	ADD liquid ingredients and mix with above to form a moderately stiff batter. Drop by large spoonfuls onto greased cookie sheet. Bake at 350° for 15 minutes. Serve with applesauce and syrup, or plain with butter.

1 dozen

Breakfast Ideas

VANDEMAN BREAKFAST

3 slices toasted whole wheat bread	LIGHTLY coat with margarine (if desired).
¼ cup peanut butter (George Vandeman prefers chunky)	STIR in water, a tablespoon at a time, and gradually whip until the consistency of whipped cream. Spread on toast.
2 or 3 cups applesauce

SERVES: 2 | HEAT applesauce and smother toast. You may find it difficult to stop with one piece! Eaten with a glass of non-fat milk, and a liberal serving of another fruit, this is a wholesome alternate to an average American breakfast. The Vandemans enjoy this breakfast at least three times a week! |

GRANOLA

157 Cal. per ½ cup

1 large box quick oats
(2 lbs. 10 oz.)
2 cups shredded coconut
2 cups wheat germ
1 cup whole wheat flour
1 Tbsp. salt
1 cup cashews (raw) or
almonds, chopped

MIX together first six ingredients.

½ cup brown sugar
¾ cup oil
1 cup honey
¾ cup water
1 Tbsp. vanilla

WHIZ together in blender. Add to dry mixture above, stirring thoroughly. Bake at 250°, stirring every 20 minutes, for about 1 hour, or until brown.

YIELD: 24 cups cereal

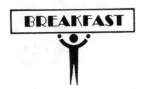

APRICOT RAISIN GRANOLA

181 Cal. per ½ cup

5 cups raw oats, quick or regular	HEAT in an ungreased pan in a 350° oven for 10 minutes.
1/3 cup brown sugar **½ cup wheat germ**	ADD to oats and mix well.
1/3 cup oil **¼ cup honey** **¼ tsp. almond extract**	COMBINE and mix with dry ingredients. Mix until dry ingredients are well coated. Bake in shallow pans at 250° 35-40 minutes. Stir often to brown evenly.
1 cup raisins **1 cup chopped dried apricots**	ADD to granola and stir well. Let cool. Store in a tightly covered container in refrigerator.

YIELD: 8 cups cereal

FOUR GRAIN CEREAL

¼ cup whole wheat grain **¼ cup millet** **¼ cup brown rice** **¼ cup pearl barley** **3 cups water** **1 tsp. salt**	COVER grains with water and allow to soak overnight. Chopped dates or raisins may also be included. In the morning, cook cereal thoroughly. Any combination of grains can be made as long as the measurements remain the same.

SERVES 4

FRUITED MILLET CEREAL

½ cup millet **½ tsp. salt** **2 cups water**	COOK over low heat for 15 minutes.
½ cup raisins or dates **½ cup chopped pecans**	ADD to cereal and continue cooking another 15 minutes. Serve with milk.

SERVES 4

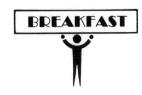

RICE CEREAL

176 Cal. per serving

1 cup brown rice, dry	PLACE in dry skillet over low flame and toast rice lightly.
2 cups water **1 tsp. salt**	PLACE rice in water and cook until tender and fluffy. Serve with chopped dates, raisins or bananas.

SERVES 4

FRUITY OATMEAL

153 Cal. per serving

1¾ cups rolled oats **4 cups boiling water** **1 tsp. salt**	SPRINKLE oats into rapidly boiling salted water. Let cook 10 minutes.
¼ cup wheat germ **10 chopped dates**	STIR in and cook on low heat 10 minutes more.
1 large banana	SLICE into oatmeal. Let stand about 2 minutes. Serve with milk.

SERVES 4

BREAKFAST OATMEAL CASSEROLE

125 Cal. per serving

4 cups cooked oatmeal **1 apple, chopped (1 cup)** **1 cup raisins** **¼ tsp. cardamom**	COMBINE and bake at 350° for 20 minutes.

SERVES 6

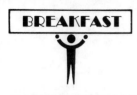

BREAKFAST

OATMEAL WAFFLES

213 Cal. per serving

4 cups quick oats
½ cup powdered milk,
   soy or skim
1 tsp. salt
3 cups hot water
¼ cup oil
sesame seeds

SERVES 6

MIX all ingredients thoroughly. Heat waffle iron and oil well for first waffle or spray with Pam before heating. Iron should be very hot before pouring in batter. Bake until brown. This waffle takes a little longer than most so don't open for at least ten minutes. The sesame seeds may be sprinkled on top before baking. Chopped nuts may also be added. After standing, if too thick, add additional water to proper consistency.

SOY WAFFLES

199 Cal. per serving

1 cup soy or dairy milk
¾ cup whole wheat flour
¼ cup soy flour
1 tsp. salt
1 Tbsp. oil
1 Tbsp. honey

2 large waffles

MIX all ingredients thoroughly and bake until brown. These waffles raise by steam and take a little longer than others. Other combinations of flour may be used for variety.

SOUTHERN JOHNNYCAKES

206 Cal. per serving

2 cups corn meal
1 tsp. salt
3 Tbsp. margarine
2 Tbsp. brown sugar
½ cup milk

2 cups boiling water.

SERVES 4

MIX all together.

ADD to make a fairly soft batter but one which will hold its shape. If too thick, add a little extra water. Drop by spoonfuls onto a hot greased griddle and flatten to ½ inch thick. Turn when brown around the edges. Serve with applesauce or syrup.

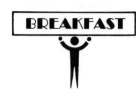

CRISPY OAT CAKES

278 Cal. per serving

1 cup water
1/3 cup oil

EMULSIFY water and oil by beating well with fork.

1 tsp. salt
1 Tbsp. honey
4 cups oatmeal
½ cup whole wheat flour
¼ cup sesame seeds

ADD and mix well. Make into balls and flatten with hands or a fork. May be rolled out and cut with a cookie cutter. Place on greased cookie sheet. Bake at 375° about 15 minutes, turning once. Serve hot or cold with fruit or applesauce.

SERVES 6

EASY CORN FRITTERS

77 Cal. per serving

1 cup drained corn kernels
3 Tbsp. corn meal
½ tsp. sugar
½ tsp. salt
1 egg, beaten

MIX all together and drop by tablespoon into deep hot oil. By deep frying quickly, they will not absorb much oil. Drain on a paper towel.

SERVES 4

COTTAGE CHEESE PANCAKES

210 Cal. per serving

1 cup cottage cheese
2 tsp. oil
¼ cup whole wheat flour
1 egg
¼ cup chopped pecans
¼ tsp. salt
1 tsp. sesame seeds

BEAT together. Drop by tablespoon onto an oiled cookie sheet. Bake at 350° for 25 minutes. Good with a fruit topping.

SERVES 4

CASHEW OAT WAFFLES

147 Cal. per serving

2 cups rolled oats
3 cups water
½ cup raw cashew nuts
2 Tbsp. whole wheat flour
2 Tbsp. oil
½ tsp. salt

COMBINE in the blender. Whiz at high speed until chopped fine and mixture is light and foamy. Let stand 10 or 15 minutes. May be refrigerated overnight if desired. Bake at high heat in waffle iron for 10 to 12 minutes.

SERVES 6

VARIATION: Sunflower seeds may be substituted for cashews.

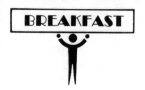

PEANUT BUTTER APPLESAUCE SPECIAL

175 Cal. per serving

4 slices whole wheat bread
2 Tbsp. peanut butter

TOAST bread in oven or automatic toaster and spread with peanut butter while warm.

2 cups applesauce

HEAT applesauce and serve hot over the toast.

SERVES 4

COTTAGE CHEESE TOAST

PLACE bread on cookie sheet.

PUT cottage cheese evenly over each slice of bread.

SPRINKLE with brewers yeast.

TOAST in oven at 350° for 15 minutes or until cottage cheese begins to melt. You may broil for a few minutes, if desired.

FRUIT TOAST

248 Cal. per serving

2 cups chopped dried fruit
2½ cups pineapple or orange juice

SIMMER fruit in juice until soft.

2 Tbsp. cornstarch
¼ cup cold water

COMBINE and add slowly to fruit, stirring constantly. Cook until thickened.

6 slices whole wheat bread

TOAST bread and pour fruit over it. The bread may be spread with peanut butter first. Try this with other fruits.

SERVES 6

SESAME TOAST

Spread whole wheat toast lightly with margarine. Invert in a plate of sesame seeds so that seeds stick to bread. Put under broiler for a few minutes, watching carefully not to burn it.

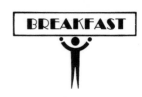
SOY OMELETTE

180 Cal. per serving

1 cup soybeans
2 cups hot water

BRING soybeans to boil, cover and remove from heat. Allow to sit one hour until softened, drain.

1½ cups water
2 Tbsp. oil
1 small onion, chopped

BLEND soaked soybeans in water with onion and oil at high speed until well pureed, 2-3 minutes.

1 Tbsp. chicken style seasoning
½ tsp. seasoned salt
½ tsp. turmeric

ADD seasonings and pour into hot oiled skillet. Stir constantly until thickened, then cover and cook slowly for 20-30 minutes until dry, stirring occasionally.

SERVES 6

CASHEW BROILER TOAST

112 Cal. per slice

1 cup raw cashews
1½ cups water
¼ cup dates
⅛ tsp. salt

BLEND nuts and dates in water.

whole wheat bread slices

SERVES 6

DIP bread slices in cashew-date milk and place on greased cookie sheet under broiler at 450° until browned. Turn and brown other side. Serve with favorite pancake topping.

GREAT NORTHERN BREAKFAST

185 Cal. per serving

1 lb. package great northern beans
6 cups water

BRING beans to a boil in kettle, then turn off heat and allow to soften for one hour. Continue cooking until tender.

1½ tsp. salt
1 cup evaporated milk

ADD salt and milk; should be soupy consistency. Serve over whole wheat toast, buttered.

SERVES 10

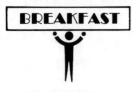

TANGY SWEET JAM

28 Cal. per Tbsp.

1 cup dried apricots **2 cups water**	SOAK overnight in water. Whiz in blender or grind in grinder.
1 cup pitted dates	ADD and continue blending or grinding until smooth.

CASHEW BUTTER

81 Cal. per Tbsp.

1 cup hot roasted cashew **nuts** **¼ cup oil**	PUT oil in blender. Add cashews gradually, while blender is running. Blend until desired consistency.

UNCOOKED MARMALADE

25 Cal. per Tbsp.

3 cups mixed, dried fruit **(prunes, apricots, peaches,** **pears, apples, etc.)**	SOAK overnight using a minimum of water. Pit prunes. Put all fruit through food grinder.
1 cup crushed pineapple	ADD and mix thoroughly.
honey	ADD to taste, if not sweet enough.

HONEY MAPLE SYRUP

58 Cal. per Tbsp.

1 cup honey	HEAT but do not boil.
1 cup pure maple syrup **1 tsp. vanilla**	ADD and stir blending well. Use sparingly.

The Two Day Kitchen Garden - Sprouts

Why sprout seed?

- Seeds are small storehouses and sprouting activates their built-in chemical laboratories to manufacture Vitamins A (if green), some of B complex, C and E
- This is the fastest way of changing nutritional value of food with a wider nutrient content
- Provides fresh greens for salads, the year around
- Inexpensive taste change for salads

What are good seed for sprouting?

Legumes: soy (mung) beans, lentils, garbanzos, peas
Grains: wheat, barley, millet, oats, rye, rice, corn
Grasses: alfalfa, sunflower

How are sprouts grown?

- Select a wide-mouthed quart jar
- One-half cup of medium-sized seed or one tablespoon of small seed will make about one quart of sprouts
- Cover seed in jar with a cheesecloth or nylon stocking lid
- Wash and rinse seed several times, then cover with water for overnight soaking
- Pour off water in morning, and rinse seed twice a day, or more often if hot weather, to keep moist. Keep bottle in dark place
- After each rinse, shake and spread seed over the bottom and side of the bottle
- Place bottle in sunlight after 48 hours to develop green color in sprouts
- Sprouts are ready to use when ¼ to ½ inch in length.

How are sprouts used?

- To replace lettuce in salads (see pgs. 125, 131)
- As a garnish for salads or soups
- To replace lettuce in sandwiches (see pg. 134)
- Sauteed (mung beans) in Chinese dishes with other vegetables (pg. 42)
- Sprouted grains in bread making (see pg. 89, 90)

SALADS

What is a fruit?

"The mature ovary of a plant or tree, including the seed, its envelope and
closely connected parts, as the pit and flesh of a peach, or a pea and
its pod." — Webster's Unabridged Dictionary

"Crops listed as fruits are usually grown on trees, shrubs, vines and fleshy-
stemmed plants. Commonly, such crops as tomatoes and melons are
classed as vegetables, although it is proper to call them vegetable fruits."
— World Book

Therefore, fruits are . . .

- Not only apples, peaches, dates, avocados, oranges, etc., (from trees)
- But pineapples, guavas, berries, etc. (shrubs)
- And seeds of plants: grains of all kinds
- And seeds of trees: nuts of all varieties
- And seeds with pods: legumes of every type
- And fruits of vines: cucumbers, squash, melons, etc.
- And fruits of fleshy-stemmed plants: tomatoes, eggplants, peppers, etc.

What, then is a a vegetable?

"In popular usage there is no exact distinction between a fruit and a vegetable,
except where the latter consists of the stem, leaves, or root of the plant."
— Webster's Collegiate Dictionary.

Therefore, vegetables are . . .

- Stems: celery, broccoli, asparagus, rhubarb, etc.
- Leaves: cabbage, lettuce, spinach, parsley, etc.
- Roots: potatoes, carrots, beets, parsnips, radishes, onion, etc.

What do fruits supply in the diet?

- Carbohydrates, proteins and fats
- Vitamins, minerals and acid
- Water and roughage, which gives laxative properties
- Sugar, which provides quick energy and endurance
- Legumes, grains and nuts are excellent sources of protein, low in fats

Vegetables are important for . . .

- Vitamins and minerals
- Good source of carbohydrates (starches)
- Bulk in diet, aiding digestion and elimination
- Most are low in calories, but help satisfy hunger
- Some protein

Salad Dressings
(Eggless)

SOYAGEN "MAYONNAISE" 55 Cal. per Tbsp.

1 cup water
½ cup Soyagen
½ tsp. salt
½ tsp. Accent
½ tsp. paprika

PLACE in blender and whiz for a few minutes.

1 cup oil

ADD to blender and whiz for several minutes.

3 Tbsp. lemon juice

REMOVE from blender and add lemon juice. This will thicken it. Refrigerate to blend flavors.

YIELD: 2½ cups

SOY TARTAR SAUCE 45 Cal. per Tbsp.

1 cup soy "mayonnaise"
1 Tbsp. minced dill pickle
1 Tbsp. minced pimento
1 Tbsp. minced onion
1 Tbsp. minced green pepper

MIX all ingredients together. Flavor improves by allowing to sit overnight.

YIELD: 1¼ cups sauce

SOYAMEL SOUR KREEM 46 Cal. per Tbsp.

1 cup water
½ cup Soyamel (powder)

BLEND the water and Soyamel in blender.

¾ cup corn oil
¼ cup lemon juice

ADD the oil slowly and then the lemon juice.

YIELD: 2½ cups

CHILL. Will keep refrigerated for 7-10 days.

SOY "MAYONNAISE" 46 Cal. per Tbsp.

1 cup Soyamel Sour Kreem
½ tsp. paprika
¼ tsp. salt
¼ tsp. onion salt
⅛ tsp. garlic salt
⅛ tsp. seasoning salt
¼ tsp. celery salt

MIX all ingredients together.

in Coleslaw

YIELD: 1 cup

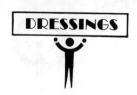

DRESSINGS

TROPICAL FRUIT DRESSING

25 Cal. per Tbsp

1 cup Soyamel Sour Kreem
½ cup crushed pineapple,
   drained
1 cup mashed bananas
¼ cup coconut, grated

MIX all together and serve on any fruit salad.

YIELD: 2½ cups

TOMATO FRENCH DRESSING

49 Cal. per Tbsp.

½ cup undiluted tomato soup
½ cup salad oil
¼ cup lemon juice
1 tsp. minced onion
½ tsp. salt
1 Tbsp. honey

MIX well and chill.

YIELD: 1½ cups

LOW CALORIE "FRENCH" DRESSING

3 Cal. per Tbsp.

1 cup tomato juice
½ cup grapefruit juice
⅛ tsp. garlic salt
dash of paprika
½ cup vegetable bouillon

MIX all ingredients well. For bouillon you may use ½ cup water with ½ tsp. of McKay's Chicken-Style Seasoning, or ½ tsp. G. Washington Broth, or ½ vegetable bouillon cube.

YIELD: 2 cups

ITALIAN DRESSING

67 Cal. per Tbsp.

1 cup salad oil
¼ cup water
½ cup lemon juice
1 tsp. salt
2 Tbsp. sugar
½ tsp. oregano
½ tsp. sweet basil
½ tsp. garlic powder
1 tsp. onion powder

BLEND together in blender until thick.

VARIATION: ½ 10 oz. can undiluted Campbell's tomato soup may be added.

YIELD: about 2 cups

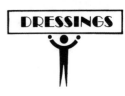

LOW CALORIE SOUR CREAM SUBSTITUTE

9 Cal. per Tbsp.

½ cup cottage cheese
½ cup buttermilk
2 tsp. lemon juice
chives, optional

OSTERIZE and serve on potatoes, etc.

YIELD: 1 cup

BOILED SALAD DRESSING

16 Cal. per Tbsp.

3 Tbsp. sugar
1 tsp. salt
1 Tbsp. flour
1 egg

MIX all together well in small saucepan.

2 Tbsp. lemon juice (or juice of
1 lemon)
½ cup water
1 Tbsp. margarine

ADD to above mixture and beat well. Cook over medium heat until thickened, stirring constantly. Cool with lid on pan. When cold, thin to desired consistency with light cream or rich milk.

YIELD: about 1½ cups

COOKED SALAD DRESSING

30 Cal. per Tbsp.

1 cup cold water or soy milk
1½ Tbsp. arrowroot powder

COOK and stir to thicken. Cool.

1 cup water
½ cup soy milk powder
¾ cup oil

MIX water and soy milk in blender. Add slowly enough oil to thicken. Add the cooled mixture.

¼ tsp. garlic powder
½ tsp. onion powder
½ tsp. celery salt
½ tsp. paprika
½ cup lemon juice
salt to taste

ADD to above mixture and blend. Refrigerate.

YIELD: 4 cups

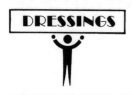

DRESSINGS

TANGY SPREAD OR DIP

57 Cal. per Tbsp.

1 cup soy "mayonnaise"
1 tsp. dehydrated onion
1 tsp. soy sauce
1 tsp. dry parsley

YIELD: 1 cup

MIX thoroughly and allow to stand at least an hour. Good on toast or crackers or as a dip for stick vegetables. Delicious on green salads.

SUNSHINE DRESSING

45 Cal. per Tbsp.

1/3 cup salad oil
1/3 cup lemon juice (about 2 lemons)
1 tsp. honey
¼ tsp. paprika
½ tsp. salt

YIELD: about 1 cup

COMBINE all ingredients in a small jar. Shake until well blended. Chill until serving time.

IMITATION MUSTARD

57 Cal. per Tbsp.

1 cup soy "mayonnaise"

PLACE in a small bowl.

2 tsp. turmeric
1 tsp. water

DISSOLVE turmeric with the water and mix well into mayonnaise.

2 tsp. onion juice
1 Tbsp. chopped parsley
1 Tbsp. lemon juice
dash of paprika
garlic and onion salt to taste

YIELD: 1¼ cups

MIX all together and refrigerate to blend flavors. The yellow color will deepen as it stands.

CONEY ISLAND SAUCE

73 Cal. per Tbsp.

½ cup water
½ cup Soyamel (Powder)

BLEND to a smooth paste.

1½ cups vegetable oil
6 Tbsp. lemon juice

ADD to blender in a smooth steady stream.

1 tsp. salt
½ tsp. Accent
¼ tsp. celery salt
¼ tsp. garlic salt
1 Tbsp. soy sauce
¼ cup onion, chopped
6 ounce can tomato paste

YIELD: 3 cups

ADD to blender. This will be quite stiff. Run blender only long enough to mix well. Refrigerate.

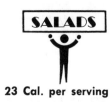

FRUIT DRESSING

23 Cal. per serving

¼ cup honey
1½ Tbsp. cornstarch

MIX in saucepan.

½ cup pineapple juice

STIR in and cook until thick stirring constantly.

2 Tbsp. lemon juice
2 Tbsp. orange juice
1 Tbsp. grated orange peel

ADD and blend in well. Cool. Serve with fruit salad.

YIELD: 1 cup

Salads

MAIN DISH TACO SALAD

252 Cal. per serving

1 large head lettuce

WASH, drain and tear into bite sizes

4 medium tomatoes, diced
2 medium onions, chopped fine

12-16 oz. mild cheddar or colby cheese

GRATE on medium sized grater

1-20 oz. can red kidney beans
2 cups meatless burger*
1 pkg. Taco flavored tortilla chips
1 cup French dressing

MIX all ingredients in large bowl. Pour over vegetables and toss lightly.

SERVES 15

ZESTY ZUCCHINI SALAD

152 Cal. per serving

3 cups thinly sliced and quartered zucchini (unpeeled)
3 large apples diced, unpeeled
½ cup diced celery
½ cup sliced water chestnuts

COMBINE zucchini, apples, celery and water chestnuts.

½ cup toasted almonds, chopped
2 Tbsp. sesame seeds

TOAST almonds, then sesame seeds in dry frying pan, turning continually until sesame seeds begin to pop or nuts lightly brown.

1 cup yogurt
2 tsp. sugar
½ cup soy "mayonnaise"
¾ tsp. salt
2 tsp. grated orange peel

COMBINE remaining ingredients in another bowl and add to zucchini mixture. Toss lightly.

SERVES 10-12

*See pg. 61

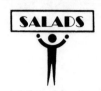

FOUR BEAN SALAD

207 Cal. per serving

2 cups cut green beans, cooked
2 cups wax beans, cooked
2 cups garbanzos, cooked
2 cups red kidney beans, cooked

COMBINE all beans, when cold.

¼ cup green pepper, diced fine
1 small onion, minced
¼ cup sugar
1/3 cup oil
1/3 cup lemon juice

COMBINE ingredients and add to beans. Salt to taste. Best if allowed to sit in the refrigerator several hours before serving.

SERVES 10

GREEN BEAN - TOMATO SALAD

96 Cal. per serving

3 cups green beans, cooked
1 small diced onion
3 cubed tomatoes
¼ tsp. salt
2-3 Tbsp. mayonnaise
pinch seasoning salt

TOSS all together. Serve immediately.

SERVES 4

CHICKEN-STYLE SALAD

131 Cal. per serving

1–10 oz. pkg. frozen lima beans (about 2 cups)

COOK, drain, and allow to cool.

2 stalks celery

CHOP fine.

½ medium onion

CHOP fine.

1 ½ to 2 cups lettuce

CHOPPED.

¼ cup mayonnaise
salt to taste

Have all ingredients chilled well. Toss thoroughly and serve on lettuce leaves, or in lettuce-lined bowl. Garnish top of salad with paprika or small slivers of pimento. Chopped pieces of chicken-style Soyameat can be added.

SERVES 6

GARBANZO SALAD

56 Cal. per serving

1 cup cooked garbanzos
¼ cup green peppers,
    chopped
2 tomatoes, chopped
1 carrot, diced
5 sprigs chopped parsley
4 celery stalks with leaves,
    chopped
1 small cucumber, chopped

MIX lightly. Add salad dressing of your choice. Pile on lettuce and garnish with radish roses.

SERVES 8

FIVE BEAN SALAD

174 Cal. per servi

2 cups green beans, cooked
2 cups wax beans, cooked
2 cups kidney beans, cooked
2 cups lima beans, cooked
1 cup bean sprouts
1 cup diced celery
1 onion, chopped
1 red pepper, diced
1 green pepper, diced

DRAIN beans and mix with celery, onions, o peppers.

½ cup sugar
2/3 cup lemon juice
½ cup salad oil
1 tsp. salt

MIX and pour over bean mixture. Let sto least 24 hours. Stir before serving.

SERVES 16

HOT PEA SALAD

73

1–10 oz. pkg. frozen peas

COOK 2-3 minutes, just u

½ cup chopped celery
¼ cup sliced green onions
1 cup diced Soyameat, turkey
    style
soy "mayonnaise" to moisten

COMBINE all ingredients
to heat through. May

SERVES 8

SALADS

MACARONI SALAD

156 Cal. per serving

1 cup dry macaroni

COOK and drain macaroni. Cool.

½ cup shredded carrot
¼ cup minced green pepper
1 cup diced celery
2 hard boiled eggs, diced
½ cup cubed cheese
2 Tbsp. onion, diced
(optional)
4 radishes, sliced (optional)

COMBINE with macaroni.

½ tsp. onion salt
4 tsp. catsup
2 tsp. lemon juice
½ cup mayonnaise
½ tsp. salt

MIX in blender and combine with macaroni mixture. Chill. Serve on lettuce leaves.

SERVES 8

PEA AND MACARONI SALAD

115 Cal. per serving

cups cooked elbow macaroni
–10 oz. pkg. frozen peas
cup finely chopped celery
small onion, minced
cup sliced, stuffed green olives
cup finely chopped green peppers
cup soy "mayonnaise"

PEAS may be used raw or half cooked.

COMBINE all ingredients with mayonnaise and serve on lettuce leaf.

VARIATION: ¼ cup slivered almonds may be added.

VES 8

OT COCONUT SALAD

125 Cal. per serving

shredded carrots
redded coconut
aisins
opped nuts, optional
neapple chunks,

pped dates,

MIX all ingredients. Use mayonnaise and salt for a dressing, or use fresh orange juice.

CAULIFLOWER TOMATO SALAD

93 Cal. per serving

1 medium cauliflower	WASH, trim and dry cauliflower.
2 tomatoes, medium **½ cup mayonnaise**	DICE tomatoes and mix with mayonnaise
	PUT cauliflower through large side of grater or cut into pieces that are chewy. Toss cauliflower lightly in the mayonnaise-tomato mixture.
SERVES 6	

MIXED CAULIFLOWER SALAD

92 Cal. per serving

1 medium raw head cauliflower, sliced thin **¼ cup minced green onion** **½ cup minced celery leaves** **½ cup chopped celery**	COMBINE cauliflower, onion, celery, and celery leaves.
½ cup sour cream **¼ cup French dressing** **1 tsp. caraway seeds** **¾ tsp. salt**	COMBINE and toss with vegetables until well blended. Serve in a bowl lined with lettuce leaves.
SERVES 6	

MARINATED ARTICHOKE HEARTS

1-10 oz. pkg. frozen artichoke hearts **1 cup water** **1 clove garlic** **juice of 1 lemon**	COMBINE in a saucepan and cook until tender, about 10 minutes. Lift artichokes out and place in a jar.
juice of ½ lemon **2 Tbsp. olive oil** **enough fluid from cooking to cover** **2 Tbsp. chopped parsley** **1 clove finely minced garlic** **SERVES 6**	ADD to cooked artichokes. Marinate overnight. Drain and use in your favorite tossed salad.

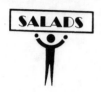

SALADS

POLISH POTATO SALAD

171 Cal. per serving

3 large potatoes

BOIL, Peel and dice

2 cups diced carrots, cooked
1 - 1 lb. can vegetarian baked beans, drained and washed
1 large onion, chopped (green onions or onion powder may be substituted)
2 hard cooked eggs, diced
2 Kosher dill pickles, chopped
1 cup celery, chopped

COMBINE all vegetables with potatoes in large bowl.

½ - 1 cup mayonnaise or as desired
2 Tbsp. lemon juice
salt to taste

STIR gently into vegetables. Refrigerate for 4-6 hours before serving.

SERVES 8-10

This is a meal in itself served with a green vegetable and whole wheat bread.

CABBAGE-POTATO SALAD

92 Cal. per serving

½ head cabbage (¾ - 1 lb.)

SHRED cabbage finely.

1 small to medium onion
4 medium, peeled, cooked potatoes
4 hard cooked eggs

DICE onion, potatoes and eggs.

mayonnaise to taste
½ tsp. salt

COMBINE all ingredients. Can mix in morning to serve at lunch. Refrigerate.

SERVES 10

CABBAGE AND GREEN LIMA BEAN SALAD

62 Cal. per serving

1 small head cabbage (shredded)
½ cup sliced radishes
½ cup finely snipped parsley
1-10 oz. pkg. frozen green lima beans
½ tsp. salt
½ can sliced onion (green tops)

MIX all ingredients. Cover and chill for one hour. Mix with sour cream and serve. Try Soy Sour Kreem, page 119.

SERVES 10

SALADS

CABBAGE AND PINEAPPLE SALAD

90 Cal. per serving

1 cup sour cream
3 Tbsp. sugar
1 tsp. salt
2 Tbsp. lemon juice

MIX together until sugar is dissolved.

3 cups finely shredded
   cabbage
1 small can crushed pineapple
   well drained. If you like
   more pineapple, a 1 lb. can
   can be used.

MIX together with the above dressing.

SERVES 10

TEBULA (LEBANESE SALAD)

309 Cal. per serving

1 cup cracked wheat
   (bulgar), dry

PLACE wheat in bowl cover with warm water
and set aside until cool. Squeeze moisture out
of wheat with hands.

4 fresh tomatoes, chopped
2 peeled cucumbers, chopped
1 medium onion, minced fine
3 heads parsley, chopped fine
1/3 cup mint flakes
2 tsp. salt
½ cup lemon juice
1 cup olive oil

TOSS wheat with chopped vegetables, salt,
lemon juice and olive oil. Refrigerate for at least
4 hours before serving. If desired, add ½ green
pepper minced fine. May substitute 4 green
onions for 1 medium onion.

SERVES 10

ONE-DISH MEAL SALAD

153 Cal. per serving

1 cup brown rice, dry
3 cups cold water
½ tsp. salt
2 Tbsp. oil

COOK rice in salted water and oil until tender.

2/3 cup diced celery
3 Tbsp. mayonnaise
1 Tbsp. French dressing
½ cup frozen peas, blanched
3 Tbsp. sweet pickle, chopped
1 tsp. onion, chopped

TOSS all ingredients together and place on
chilled lettuce-lined plates. Garnish with tomato
wedges.

SERVES 8

RAINBOW VEGETABLE SALAD

89 Cal. per serving

lettuce	ARRANGE lettuce on salad plates.
3 beets	PLACE thin slices of beets on top of lettuce in a circle.
1 cup diced carrots, cooked	ADD a circle of diced carrots.
1 cup cooked green peas	FILL the center with peas.
1 chopped green pepper	PLACE it among diced carrots.
mayonnaise	TOP with mayonnaise.

SERVES 6

CREAMY GERMAN SALAD

48 Cal. per serving

2 cucumbers, halved and thinly sliced **1 large onion, thinly sliced** **1 cup plain yogurt** **salt to taste**	COMBINE all ingredients and allow to sit for an hour or so in the refrigerator before serving. Remix.

SERVES 4

SPINACH-CUCUMBER SALAD

67 Cal. per serving

1 garlic clove	RUB salad bowl with cut garlic clove.
1 lb. fresh spinach	BREAK into bite size pieces and drain well.
½ large cucumber, partially pared	CUT cucumber into thin slices; arrange on top of spinach.
Italian Dressing, see page 120	POUR on Italian dressing, sprinkle with 1 Tbsp. lemon juice. Refrigerate. At serving time, toss, add more Italian dressing.

SERVES 6

FAVORITE SPROUT SALAD

168 Cal. per serving

2 cups alfalfa sprouts
2 cups garbanzos, cooked
2 tomatoes, diced
1 small onion, minced
½ green pepper, diced

COMBINE and toss all ingredients lightly. Good with Italian or French dressing.
(For sprouting directions, see page 117)

SERVES 4

BEET SALAD

69 Cal. per serving

1 medium head of lettuce

SHRED lettuce into 4-6 salad bowls.

1-16 oz. can shoestring beets
¼ to 1/3 cup soy "mayonnaise"

MIX well with soy mayonnaise. Place on top of lettuce.

black olives

GARNISH with black olives.

SERVES 6

HOMEMADE KOSHER DILL PICKLES

10 Cal. per pickle

3 Tbsp. pickling salt
4 cups water

COMBINE salt and water in saucepan. Bring to boil; cool.

5 to 8 cucumbers, approx. 5" long

WASH and drain cucumbers.

4 heads dill
2 cloves garlic

PUT a head of dill in the bottom of each sterilized quart jar. Pack cucumbers into jars, just to the shoulder of jar.

ADD garlic and remaining stalk of dill. Add brine to within one inch of top of jar. Adjust cap, using rubber rings and zinc caps. Store in dry, cool place 3 weeks before using.

Makes 2 quarts

RICE AND SOY CHICKEN SALAD

151 Cal. per serving

1 ½ cups diced Soyameat,
    chicken style
1 ½ cup cooked rice
1 ½ cup chopped celery
¼ cup dried onions
½ cup chopped green peppers
1 Tbsp. lemon juice
2 Tbsp. oil
¾ cup mayonnaise

COMBINE all ingredients. Can be put in a mold
and unmold to serve.

SERVES 10

SOYAMEAT STUFFED TOMATOES

171 Cal. per serving

4 tomatoes

SPOON out inside. Dice inside portion of tomato

1 - 13 oz. can Soyameat,
    chicken style, diced

DRAIN

1 stalk celery, diced
onion salt to taste
¼ cup mayonnaise

COMBINE diced tomatoes, Chix, celery, onion
salt and mayonnaise. Spoon into tomato shells.

SERVES 4

COTTAGE CHEESE STUFFED TOMATOES

130 Cal. per serving

4 tomatoes

SPOON out inside of tomatoes.

2 cups cottage cheese

SPOON ½ cup cottage cheese into each tomato.
Garnish with Baco's or Striple Zips.

SERVES 4

NUTEENA SALAD

133 Cal. per serving

2 cups cubed Nuteena
1 cup chopped celery
1-10 oz. pkg. uncooked frozen
    peas
3 Tbsp. chopped pimento
½ cup soy "mayonnaise"

MIX all ingredients together with mayonnaise
and serve on salad greens.

SERVES 8

MARINATED GARBANZO SALAD

194 Cal. per serving

2 cups cooked garbanzos,
   drained
1 medium chopped onion
4 ounces chopped pimento
¼ cup olive oil
juice of 1½ lemons
salt to taste

COMBINE all ingredients. Marinate for a few hours. Serve on crisp lettuce leaves.

SERVES 6

FRESH TURNIP SALAD

67 Cal. per serving

3 cups raw, shredded turnips
1½ cup chopped celery
2 ounces canned or chopped
   pimento
½ cup chopped or sliced ripe
   olives
¼ tsp. salt
2-3 Tbsp. mayonnaise
lettuce

COMBINE all ingredients and mix thoroughly. Serve on lettuce garnished with ripe olives, if desired.

SERVES 6

CHEESE FILLED TOMATOES

181 Cal. per serving

6 tomatoes

SPOON out inside of tomatoes.

2 cups cottage cheese (low
   fat)
1 cup shredded cheese
1/3 cup chopped olives

MIX and spoon into tomato shells.

SERVES 6

BROCCOLI SALAD

85 Cal. per serving

1 pound broccoli

COOK until just tender. Drain and chill.

3 Tbsp. olive oil
3 Tbsp. lemon juice
1 clove minced garlic
¼ tsp. salt
pimento strips

SPRINKLE over thoroughly chilled broccoli. Decorate with strips of pimento.

SERVES 6

SALADS

OPEN FACE SALAD SANDWICH
200 Cal. per serving

slice of whole wheat bread
slice of Soyameat, chicken style
1 Tbsp. soy "mayonnaise"
½ tomato, chopped
2 Tbsp. alfalfa sprouts
salt to taste

PLACE Soyameat on bread, spreading with mayonnaise. Top with tomato and sprouts. (For sprouting directions, see page 117)

PINEAPPLE WITH COTTAGE CHEESE
140 Cal. per serving

lettuce

ARRANGE on a salad plate

6 slices canned pineapple

PLACE a slice of pineapple on a lettuce leaf

cottage cheese

PLACE a scoop of cottage cheese in center of each pineapple ring

tomato

ARRANGE 1 slice of tomato in center of cottage cheese. Serve with any salad dressing, if desired.

SERVES 6

SIX CUP FRUIT SALAD
156 Cal. per serving

1 cup fresh cubed or mandarin oranges
1 cup pineapple chunks

DRAIN canned fruits thoroughly.

1 cup halved Thompson seedless grapes
1 cup banana slices
1 cup shredded or flaked coconut
1 cup plain or vanilla yogurt

COMBINE all ingredients and fold in yogurt.

SERVE on crisp lettuce leaves, if desired.

SERVES 6

WALDORF SALAD DELUXE
167 Cal. per serving

2 cups diced apples
1½ cups seeded red grapes
1 cup diced celery
½ cup coarsely chopped pecans

MIX apples, grapes, celery and pecans.

¼ cup medium cream
½ cup salad dressing
1 Tbsp. brown sugar

STIR cream, salad dressing and brown sugar till smooth. Pour dressing over apple mixture and toss lightly.

SERVES 8

HEALTH LIFESAVERS for the
Sweet Tooth . . .

Dangers in EXCESSIVE sugar intake . . .

- Obesity
- Diabetes
- Tooth Decay
- Hypoglycemia
- Elevates blood fats (triglycerides) causing arteriosclerosis
- Decreases resistance to infections
- Habit forming
- Malnutrition ("empty calories")

Sugar decreases ability of white blood cells to destroy bacteria . . .

Sugars decrease the ability of white blood cells to engulf bacteria by approximately 50%.

The greatest reduction in engulfing activity occurs about 2 hours after ingesting sugar.

Fasting increases the white cell's ability to engulf bacteria.

Therefore limiting sugar intake seems to enhance the body's defenses against infections.

Sugar content in favorite desserts or snacks . . .

Glazed Doughnut	6 tsp.	Fruit Pie (1 slice)	10 tsp.
Ice Cream (1 scoop)	4 tsp.	Canned Fruit (1 serv.)	3 tsp.
Chocolate Cake (4 oz.)	10 tsp.	Jelly or Jam (1 Tbsp.)	3 tsp.
Soft Drink (12 oz.)	8 tsp.	Gum (1 stick)	1/3 tsp.
Malted Milk (1 pt.)	15 tsp.	Banana Split	24 tsp.

Average American sugar consumption . . .

- 1822   2 teaspoons/day
- 1870   10 teaspoons/day
- 1905   20 teaspoons/day
- 1974   33 teaspoons/day

Sweet . . . but Sour

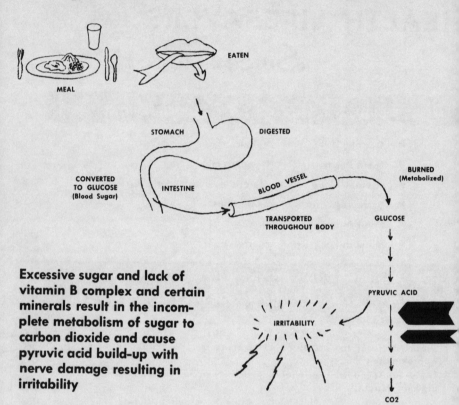

MEAL   EATEN

STOMACH   DIGESTED

CONVERTED TO GLUCOSE (Blood Sugar)   INTESTINE   BLOOD VESSEL   BURNED (Metabolized)

TRANSPORTED THROUGHOUT BODY   GLUCOSE

PYRUVIC ACID

IRRITABILITY

CO2

Excessive sugar and lack of vitamin B complex and certain minerals result in the incomplete metabolism of sugar to carbon dioxide and cause pyruvic acid build-up with nerve damage resulting in irritability

COMMON AMERICAN BREAKFAST
Coffee (no vitamins)
   Tsp. of sugar
Sweet Roll or Donut
   (sugar, little vitamins)
White Toast & Jelly
   (sugar, little vitamins)

BALANCED BREAKFAST
Fresh Fruit or Juice
Whole Grains
Protein Foods
Milk

References:
1. Sanchez, A., et al., Role of Sugars in human neutrophililic phagocytosis. Am. J. of Clin. Nut. 26: Nov. 1973
2. Scharffenberg, J. A., Special Topics in Nutrition, Book I.

Desserts

PEANUT BUTTER COOKIES

122 Cal. per cookie

½ cup peanut butter
½ cup honey
¼ cup oil
¼ tsp. salt
½ tsp. vanilla

CREAM together.

1 cup whole wheat or white
    pastry flour
4 Tbsp. wheat germ or flour

ADD and mix in. Form into flat cookies. Bake at 350° for 10 minutes. Let cool on cookie sheet before removing.

YIELD: 1½ dozen

OATMEAL COOKIES FOR A CROWD

96 Cal. per cookie

4 cups oatmeal, dry
4 cups whole wheat flour
1 cup sugar
1 cup pecan meat or walnuts
1¾ cups oil

COMBINE.

1½ cups water
1 cup powdered milk, soy or
    dairy
½ cup sorgum or molasses
½ tsp. salt
4 tsp. vanilla

BLEND and add to first mixture.

2 cups raisins
2 cups walnuts, chopped

ADD and mix well. Drop from teaspoon onto ungreased cookie sheet, flatten. Bake in 325° oven for 20 minutes.

YIELD: 8 dozen

CAROB DIAMONDS

128 Cal. per cookie

2 Tbsp. carob powder
½ cup oil
½ cup brown sugar
2 eggs
½ cup flour
¼ tsp. salt
½ tsp. vanilla

COMBINE all ingredients and mix well. Spread in two greased 8'' square pans or on cookie sheet.

½ cup chopped nuts

SPRINKLE on top of dough. Bake at 400° about 12 minutes. Cool slightly. Cut in diamonds.

YIELD: 1½ dozen

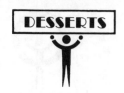

DESSERTS

SKILLET COOKIES

47 Cal. per cookie

1 cup chopped dates 1/3 cup water	COMBINE in skillet and cook over medium heat until dates are softened and the mixture is sticky.
½ cup chopped nuts	ADD and mix well. Remove from heat.
About 2 cups cereal flakes	STIR in enough dry cereal to give the desired consistency.
Coconut	SHAPE with fingers and roll in coconut.

YIELD: 2 dozen

DATE COOKIES

71 Cal. per cookie

½ cup oil 1½ cups chopped dates 1 tsp. vanilla 1 tsp. salt 1 cup whole wheat flour 1 cup rolled oats 1 cup wheat germ ½ cup liquid, milk, water or fruit juice	MIX all ingredients in order given. Nuts or raisins may be added if desired. Bake on greased cookie sheets at 350° about 15 minutes.

YIELD: 4 dozen

DANISH TYPE PASTRY TARTS

80 Cal. per tart

1 cup margarine 1 cup cottage cheese	CREAM together.
2 cups flour	MIX in to form a dough. Wrap in waxed paper and chill in refrigerator. Roll chilled dough in thin sheets. Cut out 72 rounds with a 2" cookie cutter. You may use other sizes.

¾ cup filling; may be pre-
    serves, date butter or other
    fruit
	PLACE 1 tsp. filling on half the rounds. Cover with remaining rounds and pinch together to form tarts and seal in filling. You may make large tarts by cutting dough into 18 squares, placing fruit in center, and folding over to form triangles. Bake at 400° for 15 minutes.

YIELD: 3 dozen

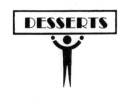

FILLED OAT CRISPS

65 Cal. per crisp

1 cup ground raisins or figs
2 Tbsp. honey
1 Tbsp. margarine
½ cup water or orange juice
1 Tbsp. grated orange rind

COOK about 5 minutes until it makes a pasty filling. Let cool while preparing dough.

1 cup margarine
½ cup brown sugar
½ tsp. salt
1 tsp. vanilla

CREAM until fluffy.

2½ cups oatmeal, dry
2½ cups whole wheat or
    white pastry flour
½ cup water or orange juice

ADD the dry ingredients alternately with the liquid. If you do not have whole wheat pastry flour, sift 3 times to remove coarser grain. Chill the mixture. Roll out a portion and cut with round cookie cutter. Place teaspoon of filling on half the rounds and place the other rounds on top. Press together with a fork around the edges. Bake at 350° until brown.

YIELD: 4 dozen

FRUIT BARS

135 Cal. per bar

½ cup coarsely chopped
    prunes
½ cup coarsely chopped
    apricots
½ cup raisins

COVER with water and cook 15 minutes. There should be about ½ cup water left. Drain the liquid to measure ½ cup and put in a bowl.

½ cup margarine
½ cup honey

CREAM with the fruit liquid.

1¼ cups sifted flour
1 cup oatmeal, dry

ADD and blend until mixture has a coarse crumb texture. With the back of a spoon firmly and evenly pack half the crumb mixture into a greased 9x9 pan. Spread filling over firmly packed crumbs. Cover with remaining half of crumb mixture making sure that all of the filling is covered. Bake at 400° for 30 minutes. Cool thoroughly before cutting in squares. Store in refrigerator.
VARIATION: Add a layer of sliced banana to the filling.

YIELD: 20 squares

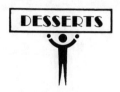

DESSERTS

CRUNCHIES

77 Cal. per square

½ cup margarine

MELT.

¼ cup honey
¼ cup sugar

ADD to melted margarine.

4 cups oatmeal, dry

ADD oats quickly before sugar dissolves completely. Blend well and press into a buttered 9 x 13 pan. Bake at 400° for 8 to 10 minutes. Cut into squares while still warm but don't remove from pan until cool.

YIELD: 2 dozen

GRANOLA COOKIES

77 Cal. per cookie

1 cup margarine

MELT.

½ cup honey
1 cup whole wheat flour
1 egg, optional
1 cup coconut
½ cup chopped nuts
3 cups oatmeal, dry

ADD ingredients in order, mixing well. Drop by teaspoon onto a greased cookie sheet. If no egg is used, press together before taking off spoon. Bake at 350° for 10 minutes. They usually bake better with 5 minutes on the top rack and 5 minutes on the bottom rack.

YIELD: 4 dozen

WHOLE WHEAT SWEET WAFERS

50 Cal. per wafer

½ cup brown sugar
6 Tbsp. vegetable shortening

CREAM together.

1 tsp. salt
¾ cup ground pecans
2 cups whole wheat flour
½ cup cold water

ADD all ingredients and mix well. Roll out thin to about ⅛ inch thickness. Cut with a pastry wheel in squares or diamonds. Bake on greased cookie sheet at 325° for 20 minutes.

YIELD: 4 dozen

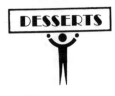
DATE SQUARES

70 Cal. per square

3 cups oatmeal, dry
1 cup flour
½ tsp salt

COMBINE oats, flour and salt.

½ cup oil

ADD and mix as for pie crust.

1 tsp. vanilla
3 Tbsp. water or milk

ADD and mix. Pat thin layer in bottom of pan (10x12). Cover with date filling (below); use last half of the mixture to cover date filling. Press down. Bake 350° for 35 minutes. Cut into squares. Let cool before removing from pan.

YIELD: 4 dozen

FILLING FOR DATE SQUARES

3 cups dates, pitted and diced
2 cups water
⅛ tsp. salt

COOK dates and water until mushy and soft and water is evaporated.

DATE-BANANA COOKIES

68 Cal. per cookie

2 large mashed bananas
1 cup chopped dates
2/3 cup oil
½ cup nuts, chopped
½ tsp. salt
1 tsp. vanilla
¼ cup soy flour
1 cup wheat germ
2 cups oatmeal, dry
¼ cup of honey

MIX all together and let stand a few minutes. Shape into cookies. Bake at 375° for 25 minutes.

YIELD: 4 dozen

FILBERT CRESCENTS

95 Cal. per cookie

1 cup margarine
¼ cup sugar

CREAM until light.

2 cups sifted flour
1 cup ground filberts
1 tsp. vanilla

ADD and mix well. Chill dough in refrigerator until firm. Shape into small crescents. Bake on ungreased cookie sheet about 10 minutes at 350°.

YIELD: 3 dozen

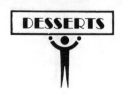

HONEY PECAN COOKIES

116 Cal. per cookie

½ cup honey
1 cup soft margarine
2 tsp. vanilla
2 cups flour
½ tsp. salt
½ cup wheat germ
1½ cups finely chopped nuts

YIELD: 3 dozen

MIX all ingredients in order given until well blended. Chill batter several hours or overnight. Form into small balls. Bake on greased cookie sheet at 325° until light brown.

THREE FRUIT PIE

263 Cal. per serving

1 cup raw cranberries
1½ cups raw apples

½ cup crushed pineapple, drained
¾ cup sugar

1 - 9" baked pie shell

Whipping cream or low-fat topping

SERVES 6

WASH, quarter, core, but do not peel apples. Put cranberries and apples through food chopper.

COMBINE with pineapple and sugar. Refrigerate 12-24 hours so that flavors blend; tastes like strawberries. Fill pie shell just before serving and top with whipped topping. Slices out beautifully —no cooking, no gelatin; just delicious raw fruit.

LOW FAT TOPPING

9 Cal. per Tbsp.

1/3 cup ice water
1/3 cup nonfat dry milk

2 Tbsp. sugar
2 Tbsp. lemon juice

YIELD: 1½ cups

MEASURE water and milk into 1 quart mixing bowl. Beat until stiff.

ADD sugar and lemon juice gradually, beating constantly. Chill ½ hour before serving.

SOYAMEL TOPPING

81 Cal. per Tbsp.

2 Tbsp. Soyamel
¼ cup water

½ cup oil, plus 1 Tbsp.
1-2 Tbsp. lemon juice
1 to 3 Tbsp. sugar or honey

MIX in blender.

ADD.

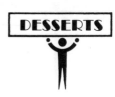

BANANA CASHEW CREAM PIE

263 Cal. per serving

1 cup water
½ cup raw cashew nuts or
    blanched almonds
12 pitted dates
1 tsp. vanilla
pinch of salt
3 Tbsp. cornstarch

BLEND ingredients in blender.

1 cup water

ADD and put in double boiler. Cook until thick.

SLICE layer of bananas into baked pie shell.
ADD cashew filling.
GARNISH with strawberries, cherries or coconut.

SERVES 6

WHOLE WHEAT PIE CRUST

¼ cup oil
3 Tbsp. water

BEAT oil and water together with fork until creamy.

1 cup whole wheat pastry
    flour
½ tsp. salt

MIX flour and salt in bowl. Pour oil-water mixture over it and knead a little. PRESS out thin between waxed paper. In pie plate, perforate bottom and sides of crust with fork. Bake at 350° for 15 minutes.

PINEAPPLE DELIGHT PIE

254 Cal. per serving

2½ cups pineapple juice
sections of 2 oranges
    (optional)
¼ - 1/3 cup cornstarch

WHIZ together in blender. Cook until thick, stirring constantly.

1 or 2 large bananas

SERVES 6

SLICE bananas or dates to cover bottom of baked pie shell. Pour slightly cooled mixture over fruit. Garnish with shredded coconut (optional) and mandarin sections.

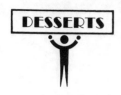

SQUASH PIE (Eggless)

219 Cal. per serving

4 Tbsp. flour	BROWN lightly stirring constantly.
½ cup brown sugar 2 cups cooked winter squash, mashed	COMBINE sugar and flour and add to squash.
½ tsp. salt 2 Tbsp. molasses ½ tsp. vanilla 1 ½ cups evaporated milk ½ tsp. cardamom	ADD to squash and mix well. You may use reconstituted powdered milk, double strength instead of the evaporated. Pour into an unbaked 9 inch pie crust. Bake at 450° for 10 minutes. Reduce heat to 325° and bake 30 to 40 minutes more until set and light brown.
	VARIATION: This recipe is good substituting pumpkin or sweet potato for the squash.

SERVES 6

HONEY APPLE PIE IN OATMEAL CRUST

287 Cal. per serving

CRUST

¼ cup soft margarine 1 Tbsp. honey	CREAM together.
¼ cup whole wheat flour ¼ tsp. salt 1 ¼ cups quick oats	MIX add to margarine. Mix well. Press over bottom and sides of a 9 inch pie pan. Bake at 375° about 15 minutes until delicately brown.

FILLING:

½ cup honey	BRING to a boil.
⅛ tsp. cardamom ⅛ tsp. coriander, optional 5 cups thinly sliced apples	ADD and cook slowly until apples are transparent. Cool. Pour into baked, cooled oatmeal crust.
½ cup whipped low calorie topping	GARNISH top.

SERVES 6

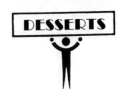
EASY PIE CRUST

1 cup unbleached enriched
    white flour
1 cup sifted whole wheat flour
1 tsp. salt

RESIFT flour and salt together.

½ cup oil
½ cup ice water

BEAT with a fork until emulsified. Pour over flour all at once, tossing lightly to mix. Form quickly into a ball, handling as little as possible. Divide in half and roll out each half between sheets of waxed paper or heavy plastic. Remove top paper and fit loosely into pie pan. For single baked crust, prick bottom and bake at 450° for 10-12 minutes.

BLUEBERRY PIE

289 Cal. per serving

4 cups blueberries

RINSE and drain in a colander.

¼ cup sugar
3 Tbsp. cornstarch
⅛ tsp. salt

MIX in a saucepan.

½ cup cold water

STIR in cold water. Add 2 cups of the berries. Cook over low heat, stirring constantly until thick. Remove from heat.

2 Tbsp. margarine
1 tsp. grated lemon rind,
    optional
1 Tbsp. lemon juice

ADD and stir. You may taste to adjust to your liking for sweetness.

1 baked pie crust, 9 inches

PUT remaining 2 cups of berries in bottom of pie crust. Cover with cooked blueberries. Cool. Garnish with whipped topping.

SERVES 6

COCONUT PIE CRUST

1/3 cup margarine
2 cups shredded coconut

COMBINE in skillet. Cook over low heat, stirring frequently until coconut is toasted and golden brown. Press into a 9 inch pie plate to form crust. Chill until firm.

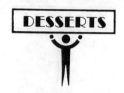

DESSERTS

PRUNE PINEAPPLE DESSERT

1-12 oz. box pitted prunes — CUT in fourths. Cover with water and simmer until soft. Drain juice and add water to make 1 cup.

1-20 oz. can unsweetened crushed pineapple
1 pkg. Danish Dessert, raspberry-currant flavor — COMBINE with the 1 cup reserved liquid and cook over medium heat until thickened and clear. Let boil 1 minute.

1 cup chopped walnuts
1 Tbsp. lemon juice
pinch of salt — COMBINE with all above ingredients and mix well. Pour into 8x13 pan. Chill several hours or overnight. Cut in squares and serve with whipped topping if desired. Mixture will be of rather soft consistency.

SERVES 12 to 15

CARROT-ORANGE CAKE

188 Cal. per serving

4 eggs
½ tsp. salt
¼ cup hot water — SEPARATE eggs, putting whites into small bowl and yokes into large bowl. Add the salt to the yolks. Beat yolks until thick adding the hot water while beating.

1 Tbsp. lemon juice — ADD to yolks.

1/3 cup oil — ADD slowly to yolks beating continuously.

½ cup sugar — ADD gradually, beating continuously.

1 cup grated raw carrot
½ cup orange juice
1 Tbsp. grated orange rind
1½ cups sifted whole wheat flour — COMBINE carrots, orange juice, and rind, and add alternately with whole wheat flour, folding gently.

1 cup coconut — FOLD in gently.

¼ cup sugar — BEAT reserved egg whites until stiff, adding sugar. Fold carefully into the batter. Use a wire whip if you have one.

½ cup chopped pecans — SPRINKLE half the nuts on bottom of tube pan, or other type. Pour batter over nuts. Sprinkle remaining nuts on top. Bake at 325° about 1 hour. Let stand 5 minutes then invert to cool. Glaze if desired.

SERVES 16

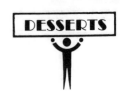

WHOLE WHEAT HONEY MOLASSES CAKE
202 Cal. per serving

3 eggs **¼ tsp. salt**	SEPARATE the eggs. Place the whites in a large bowl and yolks in a medium bowl. Add salt to whites and beat stiff, but not dry.
½ cup honey **¼ cup molasses**	WARM together in a small saucepan and add slowly to egg whites, beating until mixture stands in high peaks.
¼ tsp. salt **3 Tbsp. boiling water**	ADD to egg yolks and beat until thick and light. light.
½ cup oil	ADD gradually, beating in thoroughly. Combine the yolk and white mixture by folding carefully together.
1 ¼ cups whole wheat pastry flour	SIFT the flour over this mixture about 2 tablespoons at a time, folding it in carefully.
1 tsp. vanilla	ADD and fold in. Pour batter in a greased flat pan or deep pie plate or ungreased tube pan. Bake at 325° for 30 minutes. Tube pan takes a little longer. This cake must be thoroughly baked as it is very moist. Serve plain, or with powdered sugar sifted on top or with whipped topping.

SERVES 12

WHOLE WHEAT HONEY BANANA CAKE

Use the above recipe, substituting a mashed banana for the molasses, beating it into the whites after the honey has been beaten in. Then use ¼ cup more flour.

EASY APPLE CRISP
182 Cal. per serving

6 large apples **2 Tbsp. honey**	PEEL and slice into a baking dish. Sprinkle with honey. Cover and bake at 350° until soft.
1 ½ cups granola	SPRINKLE evenly on top. If your granola doesn't have nuts, sprinkle a few on top. Return to oven for 5 minutes. Serve plain or with whipped topping.

SERVES 6

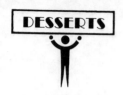

BLUEBERRY RICE SUPREME

119 Cal. per serving

2 cups boiled cooled rice (1
    cup uncooked)
½ cup flaked coconut
1/3 cup chopped walnuts
1 ½ cups fresh blueberries

MIX together and fold in low fat topping,
just before serving. (See page 142)

SERVES 8

POLYNESIAN BARS

79 Cal. per bar

¾ cup whole wheat flour
¾ cup unbleached enriched
    white flour
1 ½ cups oatmeal, dry
¾ cup soft margarine
½ cup coconut
½ cup chopped nuts

MIX all together with the hands. This will make
a crumb mixture. Press half of crumb mixture into
a greased 9 x 12 baking pan.

4 cups chopped dates
2 cups crushed pineapple,
    undrained
¾ cup water
1 tsp. vanilla

COOK filling until thick and smooth. Spread on
the crust in the pan clear to the edge. Spread the
remaining crumbs on top and pat down well.
Bake at 350° for 30 minutes. Cool and cut in
squares.

YIELD: 4 Dozen

TUTTI FRUITTI ICE KREEM

284 Cal. per cup

¾ cup soy "milk" powder
1 cup water
½ cup brown sugar
½ cup oil

LIQUIFY in a blender.

1 tsp. vanilla
pinch of salt
½ cup water
1 cup coconut milk or milk
2 thoroughly mashed bananas
1 cup crushed pineapple
¼ cup red cherries, chopped

ADD. Freeze in an Ice Cream Freezer.

YIELD: 2 quarts

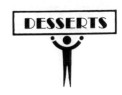

DELICIOUS, THICK BANANA SHAKE

202 Cal. per serving

4 bananas

PEEL, cut each banana into 4 pieces and freeze.

1 quart water
1½ cups soy "milk" powder
4 Tbsp. carob powder
¼ cup honey
¼ tsp. vanilla

BLEND these five ingredients and pour half of the liquid into a refrigerator tray to freeze.

TO MAKE SHAKE: Whiz in blender half of liquid, half of frozen mixture and 2 frozen bananas at a time; then repeat with remaining mixture and bananas.

SERVES 8

VARIATION: Use 1½ cups carob flavored soyagen instead of plain and omit carob powder.

FROZEN FRUIT SALAD

154 Cal. per serving

1 can, (about 2 cups) fruit
cocktail (juice and all)
1 can (about 2 cups)
crushed pineapple
1 - 6 oz. can frozen orange
juice
1 orange cut into segments
3 large bananas, sliced
1 apple, chopped

MIX together and freeze in tall plastic container or milk carton. To serve, cut in slices after running hot water over container to loosen fruit.

SERVES 10

MINTED PINEAPPLE SLUSH

102 Cal. per ½ cup

1-16 oz. can pineapple chunks
or crushed pineapple
a few sprigs of fresh mint

WHIZ in blender until smooth. Freeze until slushy. Break up with fork and spoon into dessert dishes. Number of servings depend on can size you use.

FRUITY SHERBERT

121 Cal. per serving

1 ripe banana
1-6 oz. can undiluted frozen
orange juice
1-1 lb. can crushed pineapple
½ cup powdered milk

WHIZ in blender until smooth. Pour into freezer tray and freeze until mushy. Whip with egg beater and return to freezer until firm.

SERVES 8

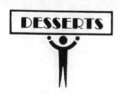

DESSERTS

CHEESE EMPANADAS

56 Cal. per cookie

¾ cup margarine
¼ cup boiling water
1 Tbsp. milk

COMBINE in bowl and whip together with a fork to emulsify.

2 cups flour
1 tsp. salt

SIFT together into the shortening mixtu·e. Stir quickly until dough cleans bowl. Roll out into 3 inch circles using additional flour as necessary.

1 lb. small curd cottage cheese FILL each circle with about 1 tsp. of cheese.

sugar
cinnamon, optional

SPRINKLE lightly with sugar and cinnamon if desired. Fold dough over to form crescent. Pinch end together. Sprinkle with additional sugar. Bake on ungreased cookie sheet at 400° about 30 minutes or until browned. For fruit empanadas fill with thickened fruit or preserves.

YIELD: 3 dozen

FRUIT SOUP

132 Cal. per serving
(without topping)

2½ cups pineapple juice
3 Tbsp. Minute Tapioca

COOK until thick.

½ cup raisins
1 diced apple
1 cup sliced peaches
1–10 oz. pkg. frozen straw-
berries

ADD. Chill until ready to serve.

sliced bananas
whipped topping

Garnish with sliced bananas and whipped topping.

SERVES 8

JOHNNY APPLESEED RICE PUDDING

167 Cal. per serving

½ cup brown rice, dry
2 cups apple juice
⅛ tsp. salt
1 Tbsp. margarine
2 Tbsp. raisins

COMBINE and bring to a boil. Cover and cook on low heat for 40 minutes.

1½ cups diced apples
2 Tbsp. honey

ADD and cook 10 minutes longer. Top with nuts and serve plain or with cream or whipped topping.

SERVES 6

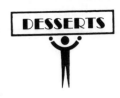

FRUIT NUT SQUARES

59 Cal. per square

¼ cup honey

HEAT almost to boiling.

½ cup dates
½ cup raisins
½ cup dried apricots
1 cup nuts

GRIND and add to warm honey.

¼ cup wheat germ

STIR in and spread in a buttered pan. Chill till firm. Cut in square.

YIELD: 30 pieces

FIG WALNUT BARS

69 Cal. per bar

1 cup dried figs
1 cup raisins
1 cup walnuts

GRIND or chop fine all ingredients. Press in thin layers and cut in strips about 4 inches long and 1 inch wide. Wrap in waxed paper and chill.

YIELD: 2 dozen

CAROB FUDGE

89 Cal. per piece

½ cup soft margarine
½ cup honey

CREAM together.

½ cup carob powder

ADD and cream well.

¾ to 1 cup soy "milk" powder

ADD enough milk powder so that the mixture is not too sticky to roll.

nuts
coconut

ROLL balls in nuts or coconut or add nuts to mixture and roll in coconut. Refrigerate to firm. Placing them in the freezer makes this especially good and chewy.

YIELD: 2 dozen

PECAN SANDIES

95 Cal. per piece

1 cup margarine
1 cup finely chopped pecans
4 Tbsp. powdered sugar
2 cups sifted flour
½ tsp. salt
1 tsp. vanilla

SOFTEN margarine and combine ingredients in order. Mix thoroughly. Form into balls or crescents. Bake slowly in a 300° oven until golden brown.

YIELD: 3 dozen

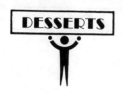

DESSERTS

NO BAKE ROLLED OAT CLUSTERS

64 Cal. per piece

¾ cup honey ½ cup margarine ⅛ tsp. salt	COMBINE in a saucepan and bring to a full boil. Remove from heat.
1 tsp. vanilla 1 cup peanut butter	ADD and stir until smooth.
3 cups oatmeal, dry YIELD: About 4 dozen	ADD and mix well. Cool slightly. Drop by tablespoons on waxed paper. Chill. When cool may be rolled in coconut or chopped nuts.

NO BAKE CAROB BALLS

33 Cal. per ball

¼ cup margarine ½ cup honey ½ cup grated apples or applesauce 2 Tbsp. carob powder ¼ tsp. salt	COMBINE in a saucepan and boil for one minute. Remove from heat.
1½ cups oatmeal, dry ½ cup chopped nuts ½ tsp. vanilla	Stir quickly into hot mixture. Mix thoroughly and drop heaping teaspoonfuls on waxed paper.
coconut YIELD: 4 dozen	ROLL in coconut when cool.

TAHINI HALVAH

1 cup sesame tahini ¼ cup honey	CREAM together until smooth.
¾ - 1 cup soy "milk" powder	ADD enough soy milk powder to make it stiff.
nuts (optional) YIELD: 2 dozen	PACK into a pan and press chopped nuts on top if desired. Harden in refrigerator. Slice and serve.

Index

INDEX

INDEX

Recommended Reading

375 Meatless Recipes–CENTURY 21   *Ethel Nelson MD* $7.95
This book will help you learn how to feed your family in such a way that
they will enjoy eating the foods that nutritionists tell us are an absolute
must if we are going to make it into the twenty-first century.

INCREDIBLE EDIBLES   *Eriann Hullquist* $7.95
What's for dinner? If you're asked this and don't have an answer, this
book is for you. A four week planner with great tasting vegetarian recipes!

CARING KITCHENS RECIPES   *Gloria Lawson* .... $ 12.95
This cookbook specializes in recipes for better health that feature: whole
grains, vegetarian, dairy free and nourishing desserts.

NUTRITION WORKSHOP GUIDE   *E. Hullquist* ... 10 for $9.95
The Nutrition Workshop Guide was developed as a handout for nutrition,
health and cooking schools to help those who are desiring to improve their
dietary life-style.

DON'T DRINK YOUR MILK   *Frank Oski, MD* $5.95
Dr. Oski, who is the head of Pediatrics at Johns Hopkins University
School of Medicine gives the frightening new medical facts about the
world's most overrated nutrient.

WHO KILLED CANDIDA?   *Vicki Glassburn* $17.95
Although diet is an important part of getting well, even the best food and
supplements are undermined if you continue to unknowingly support yeast
growth! Vicki will show you how making simple life-style choices can ac-
tually STOP THE YEAST SUPPORT CYCLE that other Candida
programs do not address.

To order any of the above titles see you local bookstore.
If you are unable to find them, send check, money order, or
Visa/Mastercard info along with shipping and handling (USA $1.65,
Canada $ 3.30, all other countries $6.60) to:

TEACH Services
Route 1, Box 182
Brushton, New York 12916 USA

or call 1(800) 367-1844 in US/Canada
(518) 358-2125 or FAX to (518) 358-3028